Pancreatology

Founded 2001 by M.V. Singer and C.W. Imrie

AF882689

KARGER

Printed in Switzerland on acid-free paper by Reinhardt Druck, Basel

Appears bimonthly: 1 volume per year (6 issues)

Journal Reprint

An essential resource for infectiologists, gastroenterologists and digestive surgeons

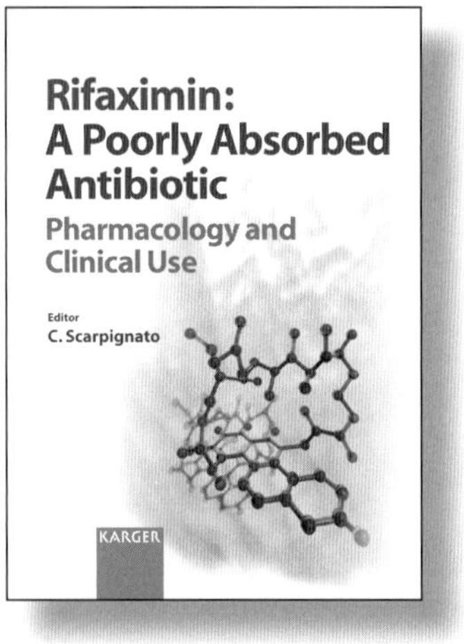

Rifaximin: A Poorly Absorbed Antibiotic

Pharmacology and Clinical Use

Editor
Carmelo Scarpignato

Pharmacology, Infectious Diseases, Gastroenterology, Digestive Surgery

Rifaximin is a semisynthetic rifamycin which is not absorbed from the gastrointestinal tract. It has been available in Europe and other countries for several years, and has recently been approved for treatment of traveler's diarrhea in the United States. Because of its broad spectrum of antimicrobial activity, rifaximin has been used with success in the treatment of infectious diarrhea, hepatic encephalopathy, small intestinal bacterial overgrowth, inflammatory bowel disease, and colonic diverticular disease. Potential indications include the irritable bowel syndrome and chronic constipation, *Clostridium difficile* infection and bowel preparation before colorectal surgery.

In this publication both the present and future clinical use of rifaximin as well as the pharmacology behind it are extensively reviewed. Compiling the latest information on this remarkably active antibacterial agent, it will be an essential resource for infectiologists, gastroenterologists, and digestive surgeons alike.

Contents

www.karger.com/rifaximin

KI 05254

Chemotherapy
Editor: Sörgel, F. (Nürnberg-Heroldsberg)
ISSN 0009–3157
Hardcover reprint: Vol. 51, Suppl. 1, 2005

Rifaximin: A Poorly Absorbed Antibiotic
Pharmacology and Clinical Use
Editor: Scarpignato, C. (Parma)
XII + 238 p., 28 fig., 5 in color, 43 tab., hard cover, 2005
CHF 98.– / EUR 70.– / USD 89.25
Prices subject to change
EUR price for Germany, USD price for USA only
ISBN 3–8055–7917–9

KARGER

Order Form

Please send: _____ copy/ies

Postage and handling free with prepayment

Payment:
☐ Check enclosed ☐ Please bill me

Please charge to my credit card
☐ American Express ☐ Diners ☐ Eurocard
☐ MasterCard ☐ Visa

Card No.: ____________________

Exp. date: ____________________

Orders may be placed with any bookshop, subscription agency, directly with the publisher or through a Karger distributor.

Fax: +41 61 306 12 34

S. Karger AG, P.O. Box, CH–4009 Basel (Switzerland)
E-Mail orders@karger.ch, **www.karger.com**

Name/Address: ____________________

____

____

____

____

Date: ____________________

Signature: ____________________

Journal Publication

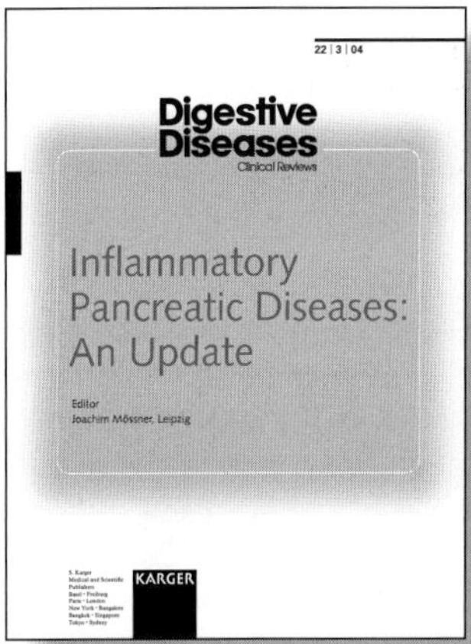

Inflammatory Pancreatic Diseases: An Update

Editor
Joachim Mössner

Gastroenterology, Molecular Biology, Pathology, Cell Biology

Contents

This publication presents new and fascinating insights especially into the pathogenesis of both acute and chronic pancreatitis. It starts with a literature review and presentation of the authors' own data on laboratory markers of acute pancreatitis such as trypsinogen, serum amyloid A and procalcitonin, paying special attention to their clinical usefulness and test performance for stratifying severity and monitoring disease progression. Also discussed is the still difficult differential diagnosis between pancreatic cancer and chronic pancreatitis, especially the early diagnosis of pancreatic cancer in preexisting chronic pancreatitis: particularly, the high specificity of molecular alterations in pancreatic cancer – as found in some pilot studies – has the potential of a strong complementary marker of malignancy in patients with a pancreatic mass of uncertain origin. Further topics discussed are acute-phase reactions during early pancreatic cellular injury, tropic pancreatitis, the pathogenesis of pain in chronic pancreatitis and the pathomechanisms of pancreatic fibrogenesis and the role of pancreatic stellate cells in the fibrotic process. Last but not least, endoscopic therapies in chronic pancreatitis are looked into.

KI 05642

www.karger.com/ddi

Digestive Diseases
Editor: Malfertheiner, P. (Magdeburg)
ISSN 0257–2753
Special issue: Vol. 22, No. 3 (2004)
Included in subscription

Inflammatory Pancreatic Diseases: An Update
Editor: Mössner, J. (Leipzig)
68 p., 14 fig., 2 in color, 7 tab., soft cover, 2004
CHF 29.– / EUR 20.50 / USD 26.50
Prices subject to change
EUR price for Germany, USD price for USA only
ISBN 3–8055–7900–4

KARGER

Order Form

Please send: _____ copy/ies

Postage and handling free with prepayment

Payment:
☐ Check enclosed ☐ Please bill me

Please charge to my credit card
☐ American Express ☐ Diners ☐ Eurocard
☐ MasterCard ☐ Visa

Card No.: ____________________

Exp. date: ____________________

Orders may be placed with any bookshop, subscription agency, directly with the publisher or through a Karger distributor.

Fax: +41 61 306 12 34

S. Karger AG, P.O. Box, CH–4009 Basel (Switzerland)
E-Mail orders@karger.ch, **www.karger.com**

Name/Address: ____________________

Date: ____________________

Signature: ____________________

General Information

Publication data: 'Pancreatology' is published 6 times a year. Volume 5 with 6 issues appears in 2005.

Subscription rates: Subscriptions run for a full calendar year. Prices are given per year.

Personal subscription:

Print or Online	Print/Online combined
CHF 563.20	CHF 604.20
EUR 417.20	EUR 447.20
USD 512.00	USD 549.00
postage and handling	(added to print and print/online)
CHF 32.70 Europe,	CHF 48.60 Overseas
EUR 23.70	
USD 44.10	

Institutional subscription:

Print or Online	Print/Online combined
CHF 1408.–	CHF 1521.–
EUR 1043.–	EUR 1127.–
USD 1280.00	USD 1383.00
postage and handling	(added to print and print/online)
CHF 40.80 Europe,	CHF 60.60 Overseas
EUR 29.40	
USD 55.20	

Airmail surcharge: CHF 40.80 / USD 33.90

Discount subscription prices:
Please enquire about reduced rates for members of affiliated societies.

Microforms: Please direct all enquiries and orders to:
University Microfilms Inc.
300 North Zeeb Road, P.O. Box 1346
Ann Arbor, MI 48106-1346 (USA)

Subscription orders: Orders can be placed at agencies, bookstores, directly with the Publisher
S. Karger AG, P.O. Box
CH–4009 Basel (Switzerland)
or with any of the following distributors:
Deutschland: S. Karger GmbH, Postfach
D–79095 Freiburg
France: Librairie Luginbühl
36, bd de Latour-Maubourg
F–75007 Paris
Great Britain, Ireland: S. Karger AG
4 Rickett Street
London SW6 1RU, UK
USA: S. Karger Publishers, Inc.
26 West Avon Road, P.O. Box 529
Farmington, CT 06085, USA
India, Bangladesh, Sri Lanka:
Panther Publishers Private Ltd.
33, First Main
Koramangala First Block
Bangalore 560 034, India
Japan: Karger Japan, Inc.
Yushima S Bld. 3F
4-2-3, Yushima, Bunkyo-ku
Tokyo 113-0034, Japan

Change of address: Both old and new address should be sent to the subscription source.

Single issues and back volumes: Information can be obtained through the Publisher.

Advertising: Correspondence and rate requests should be addressed to the Publisher.

Bibliographic indices: This journal is regularly listed in bibliographic services, including *Current Contents®*.

Book Reviews: Books are accepted for review by special agreement.

Pancreatology

Contents Vol. 5, Suppl. 1, 2005

History of the European Pancreatic Club: The First 40 Years 1965–2005

Part 1

Part 2

Abstracts

KARGER

Fax +41 61 306 12 34
E-Mail karger@karger.ch
www.karger.com

Access to full text and tables of contents, including tentative ones for forthcoming issues: www.karger.com/pan_issues

S. Karger
Medical and Scientific Publishers
Basel • Freiburg • Paris • London
New York • Bangalore • Bangkok
Singapore • Tokyo • Sydney

Drug Dosage
The authors and the publisher have exerted every effort to ensure that drug selection and dosage set forth in this text are in accord with current recommendations and practice at the time of publication. However, in view of ongoing research, changes in government regulations, and the constant flow of information relating to drug therapy and drug reactions, the reader is urged to check the package insert for each drug for any change in indications and dosage and for added warnings and precautions. This is particularly important when the recommended agent is a new and/or infrequently employed drug.

P.O. Box, CH–4009 Basel (Switzerland)
Printed in Switzerland on acid-free paper by
Reinhardt Druck, Basel
ISBN 3–8055–7993–4

KARGER

Fax +41 61 306 12 34
E-Mail karger@karger.ch
www.karger.com

Pancreatology

History of the European Pancreatic Club: The First 40 Years 1965–2005

Part 1 & 2

Authors
Harald Goebell, Essen
Rudolf Ammann, Zurich
Werner Creutzfeldt, Göttingen

Guest Editors
Thomas Griesbacher, Graz
Markus M. Lerch, Greifswald
Manfred V. Singer, Mannheim

KARGER
Basel · Freiburg · Paris · London · New York ·
Bangalore · Bangkok · Singapore · Tokyo · Sydney

Pancreatology

Pancreatology 2005;5(suppl 1):1–15
DOI: 10.1159/000086210

Published online: June 6, 2005

History of the European Pancreatic Club: The First 40 Years 1965–2005

The Development of the European Pancreatic Club as a Scientific Society

Harald Goebell[a] Rudolf Ammann[b] Werner Creutzfeldt[c]

[a]University of Essen, Essen, Germany; [b]University of Zurich, Zurich, Switzerland; [c]University of Göttingen, Göttingen, Germany

Abstract

The European Pancreatic Club (EPC) was founded during a first symposium on December 9 and 10, 1965 in London (President H.T. Howat). The nine founding members were one biochemist (Jean Christophe, Belgium), one physiologist (Alfred A. Harper, UK), two surgeons (André Delcourt, Belgium, Yngve Edlund, Norway) and five physicians with special interest in the pancreas (Werner Creutzfeldt, Germany, Oliver Fitzgerald, Ireland, Karel Herfort, Czechoslovakia, Henry T. Howat, UK, Henri Sarles, France). It was the first scientific society worldwide which was concerned with the study of the pancreas. The idea was to bring basic scientists and clinicians together in an informal atmosphere to promote friendship and communication on research between them. The 2nd symposium was held in Marseilles in1967 (President H. Sarles). Until now there have nearly always been annual meetings, the one in 2005 is the 37th. In 1973 the EPC decided to lay down 'Internal Rules' and in 1992 new statutes were introduced. It became a member of the United European Gastroenterology Federation (UEGF) and is coorganizer of the United European Gastroenterology Week (UEGW). The official journal has been *Pancreatology* since 2001; previously the abstracts had been printed in *Digestion* since 1982. The officers of the EPC are the President, the Past President, the President Elect, the Secretary, the Treasurer and six Councillors from different European countries, three from basic and three from clinical science. A selection committee (4 basic and 4 clinical scientists) decides on the acceptance of papers. Officers and Presidents are elected by the General Assembly. At the meetings on average 150 contributions are accepted for presentation; the abstracts are printed in *Pancreatology*. Papers came from nearly all European countries and from overseas. In numbers Germany, France, the UK, Italy and Sweden are at the top. In total 4,837 scientific presentations were made from 1971 to 2004. Fifty-nine symposia and 245 invited lectures informed about the state of the art. Since 1991 a Young Researchers Corner given by international experts is especially designed to give information on new techniques of research. The European Study Group of Pancreatic Cancer (ESPAC) and the European Registry of Hereditary Pancreatitis and Familial Pancreatic Cancer (EUROPAC) are affiliated with the EPC. Since 1999 a Newsletter of the EPC has been published. The website of the EPC is www.e-p-c.org.

Introduction

'Apparently, the first pancreatic society to be organised (world-wide) was the European Pancreatic Club (EPC), its initial meeting being held in London, December 9–10, 1965. It was created to foster communication between basic scientists and clinicians, approximately 50% of its membership and leadership representing each of those

KARGER

Fax +41 61 306 12 34
E-Mail karger@karger.ch
www.karger.com

1424–3903/05/0057–0001$22.00/0

Accessible online at:
www.karger.com/pan

Prof. emeritus Dr. Harald Goebell
Department of Gastroenterology and Hepatology
University of Essen, Universitätsklinikum, Hufelandstrasse 55
DE–45122 Essen (Germany)
Tel. +49 201 263355, Fax +49 201 2667393, E-Mail harald.goebell@uni-essen.de

Table 1. List of those participating in or attending the Symposium on Normal and Abnormal Functions of the Exocrine Pancreas, 30 May to 1 June, 1961, in London

V. Becker	Pathologisches Institut der Universität Kiel
J.J. Bernier	Hôpital Bichat, Paris
B. Borgström	Department of Physiological Chemistry, University of Lund
W. Burnett	Department of Surgery, Western Infirmary, Glasgow
W.I. Card	Gastro-Intestinal Unit, Western General Hospital, Edinburgh
A.M. Dawson	Department of Medicine, Royal Free Hospital, London
P. Desnuelle	Laboratoire de Chimie Biologique, Marseilles
D.A. Dreiling	Mount Sinai Hospital, New York, N.Y.
R. Ekholm	Department of Anatomy, University of Gothenburg
J.B. Gross	Mayo Clinic, Rochester, Minn.
M.I. Grossman	Section of Gastroenterology, Veterans Administration Hospital, Los Angeles, Calif.
A.A. Harper	Department of Physiology, King's College, Newcastle upon Tyne
L.E. Hokin	Department of Physiological Chemistry, University of Wisconsin, Madison, Wisc.
Mabel E. Hokin	Department of Physiological Chemistry, University of Wisconsin, Madison, Wisc.
H.T. Howat	Manchester Royal Infirmary, Manchester
J.N. Hunt	Physiological Laboratory, Guy's Hospital, London
H.D. Janowitz	Mount Sinai Hospital, New York, N.Y.
J.E. Jorpes	Kemiska Institutionen, Karolinska Institutet, Stockholm
H. Lagerlöf	Karolinska Sjukhuset, Stockholm
V. Mutt	Kemiska Institutionen, Karolinska Institutet, Stockholm
H. Neurath	Department of Biochemistry, University of Washington, D.C.
G.E. Palade	Rockefeller Institute, New York, N.Y.
H. Sarles	Faculty of Medicine, Marseilles
Sheila Sherlock	Department of Medicine, Royal Free Hospital, London
S.S. Sjöstrand	Department of Zoology, University of California, Los Angeles, Calif.
R.E. Turnbridge	Department of Medicine, General Infirmary, University of Leeds
P.V. Veghelyi	Department of Pediatrics No. 1, University Medicine School, Budapest
C.L. Vink	St. Josef Ziekenhuis, Eindhoven

two categories' [1]. In the last 4 decades at least 15 national and international organizations and 6 national or international journals which provide channels of specific communication in the limited field of pancreatology have been started [see 1]. So this small organ – the pancreas – must in many ways be fascinating to the scientific community.

Progress in the knowledge of pancreatology has developed at a slower rate than in other fields of gastroenterology. This is due in part to the difficult accessibility of the organ in humans and also for physiological studies in animals. In the past there were few scientific centers with special interest in pancreatic physiology, biochemistry and pancreatic diseases and the exchange between them was hampered by the fact that these centers were spread worldwide. With the marked progress within basic science and the rapidly increasing development of new diagnostic tools, the increased need for closer cooperation between centers in Europe and internationally in particular the exchange of recent interdisciplinary experience between 'bench' and 'bedside' became obvious.

The main purpose of the present study is to summarize the historical evolution of pancreatology based on the history of the EPC over 40 years. This has recently also been done for the Japanese Pancreas Society [2] and the American Pancreas Club [3].

The First Two European Symposia (1961, 1963) Preceding the Foundation of the EPC

In the year 1961 the Ciba Foundation in London organized a symposium on The Exocrine Pancreas: Normal and Abnormal Functions [4] (fig. 1). It followed a suggestion, which had been made by H.D. Janowitz and was under the skillful chairmanship of Sheila Sherlock. Twenty-eight specialists were invited, who represented the main centers of worldwide research on the pancreas at

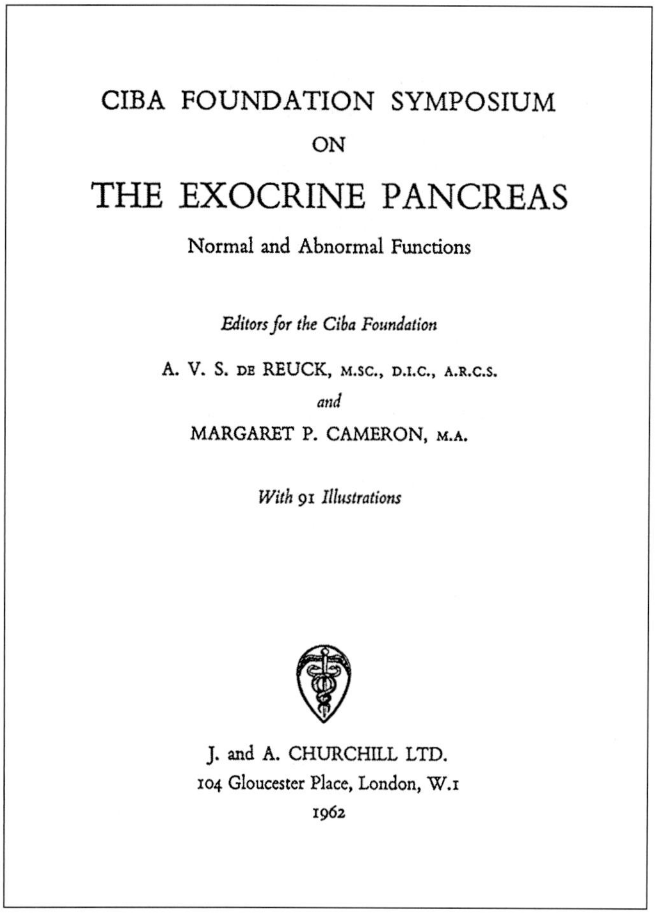
CIBA FOUNDATION SYMPOSIUM
ON
THE EXOCRINE PANCREAS
Normal and Abnormal Functions

Editors for the Ciba Foundation
A. V. S. DE REUCK, M.SC., D.I.C., A.R.C.S.
and
MARGARET P. CAMERON, M.A.

With 91 *Illustrations*

J. and A. CHURCHILL LTD.
104 Gloucester Place, London, W.1
1962

Fig. 1. Title page of the Ciba Foundation Symposium, London, 1961, published 1962.

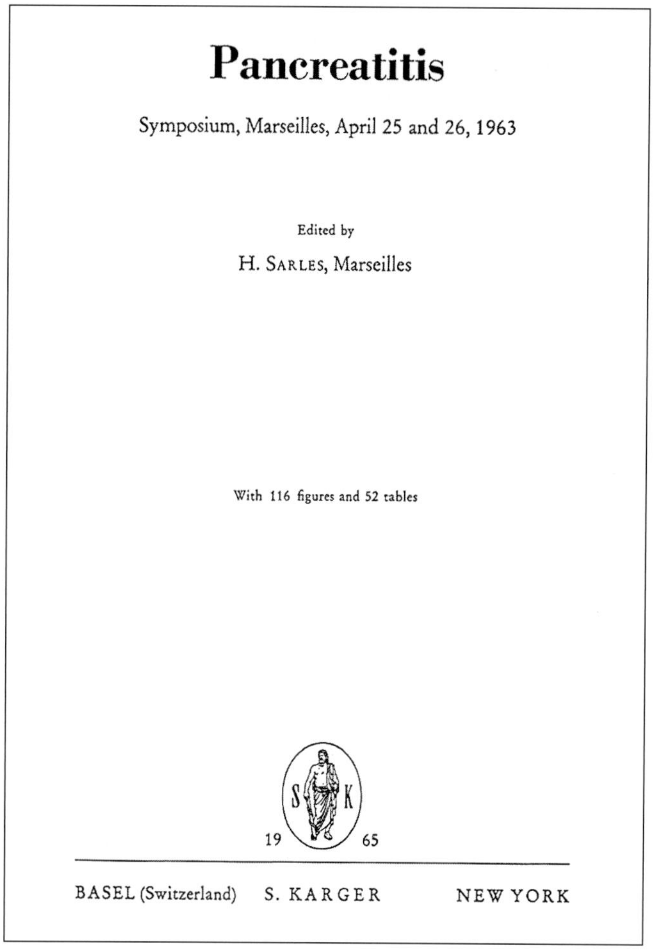
Pancreatitis
Symposium, Marseilles, April 25 and 26, 1963

Edited by
H. SARLES, Marseilles

With 116 figures and 52 tables

19 65

BASEL (Switzerland) S. KARGER NEW YORK

Fig. 2. Title page of the Marseilles Symposium on Pancreatitis, 1963, published 1965.

that time (table 1). The topics covered ultrastructure and histochemistry of the organ, the nature of pancreatic secretion, the physiological control of pancreatic secretion, the assessment of pancreatic function and the abnormal pancreas with genetic and metabolic aspects. In all these fields important progress was made in the 1950s. The work of George E. Palade had introduced electron microscopy into the study of dynamic secretory processes in the acinar cell, work that finally led to the his winning the Nobel Prize in 1974. The isolation and characterization of the gastrointestinal hormones secretin and cholecystokinin/pancreozymin by A.C. Ivy, A.A. Harper, J.E. Jorpes and V. Mutt, the refinements of research in enzymology (H. Neurath, L.E. Hokin, P. Desnuelle) and the studies of the mechanisms of secretion of electrolytes and enzymes and their regulation by hormonal and nerval control (M.I. Grossman) gave new impulses to research.

The clinical problems of pancreatic diseases were the topic of another symposium in Marseilles in 1963, which was organized by Henri Sarles [5] (fig. 2). This meeting had 23 invited participants, all clinicians, and led to the formulation of a classification of pancreatitis. The main topic of the symposium was chronic pancreatitis with all its facets from etiology and morbid anatomy to the clinical profile of this disease.

Thus, the interest in the pancreas increased steadily during these years both among basic scientists and clinicians. The pancreas was a model organ for physiologists and biochemists and stimulated clinical research in the field of acute and chronic pancreatitis and pancreatic carcinoma.

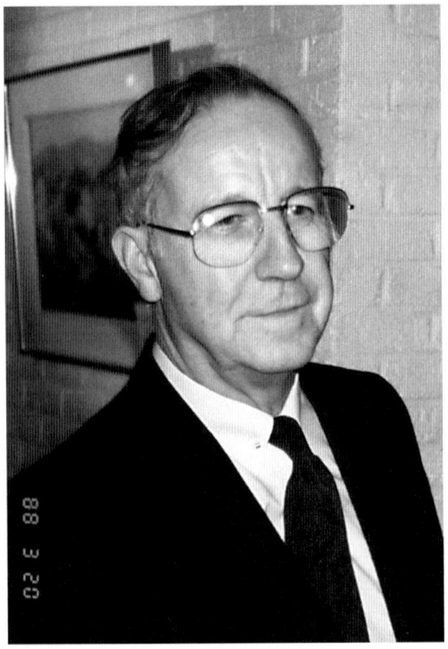

Fig. 3. Prof. A. Delcourt.

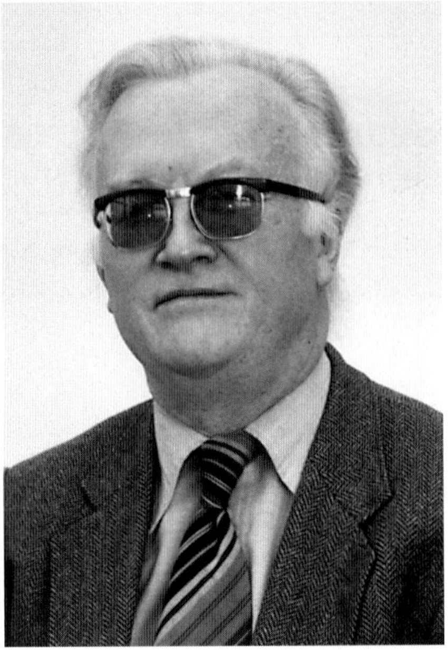

Fig. 4. Prof. J. Christophe.

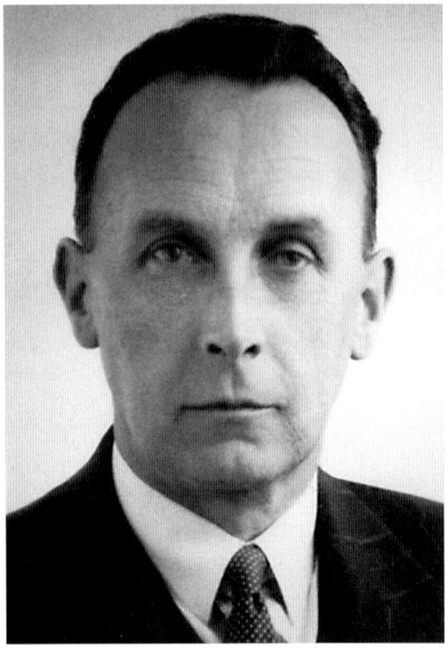

Fig. 5. Prof. A.A. Harper.

Table 2. Members of the founding meeting of the EPC in 1965

Jean Christophe	Brussels, Belgium
Werner Creutzfeldt	Göttingen, Germany
André Delcourt	Brussels, Belgium
Yngve Edlund	Gothenburg, Sweden
Oliver Fitzgerald	Dublin, Ireland
Alfred A. Harper	New Castle, UK
Karel Herfort	Prague, Czech Republic
Henry T. Howat	Manchester, UK
Henri Sarles	Marseilles, France

The Foundation of the EPC and the First Years

On December 9 and 10, 1965, again with the assistance of the Ciba Foundation, and on the initiative of Henry T. Howat and Henri Sarles, a group of nine scientists founded the EPC in London (table 2). Their portraits are given in figures 3–11. A short report, which was published by Howat [6] in *Gut* and which used the name 'European Pancreatic Club' for the first time, reveals that a group of 25 scientists and clinicians from Europe gathered in London on this occasion for a small meeting on pancreatic enzymes. This meeting in December 1965 was the founding event and actually the first symposium of the EPC. The idea was to create a platform for the exchange of information and ideas and to promote friendship between basic and clinical scientists in Europe who have a special interest in the study of exocrine function or disease.

In the first years the founding members served on a kind of 'Council'. There were no statutes and no formal regulations.

On April 28 and 29, 1967 Henri Sarles organized the second symposium of the EPC in Marseilles (Deuxième Colloque Européen du Pancréas [7]). Thirty-four papers were presented in English, French or German. A major part of the papers were dedicated to basic sciences, pathology and pathophysiology, and a special section dealt with radiological methods, mainly angiography of the pancreas. The effect of alcohol was of special interest and the pathophysiology of acute pancreatitis was also investigated. The abstracts of the presented papers were published in the *Archives Françaises des Maladies de l'Appareil Digestif* [7]. This revealed that there was really an interest among European basic and clinical scientists in the pancreas, and the success of the meeting demonstrated that there was a critical mass large enough to have a fruitful exchange at special meetings.

The third symposium of the EPC took place in 1968 in Prague under the presidency of Karel Herfort. It oc-

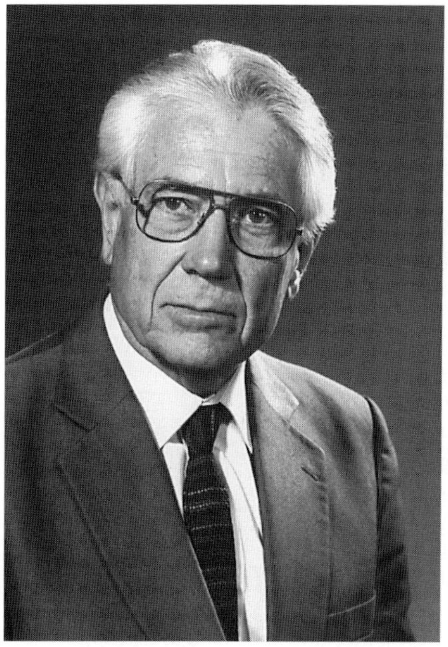

Fig. 6. Prof. H. Sarles.

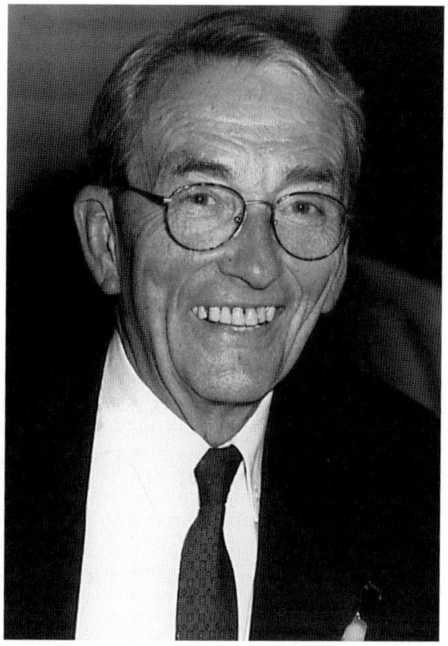

Fig. 7. Prof. W. Creutzfeldt.

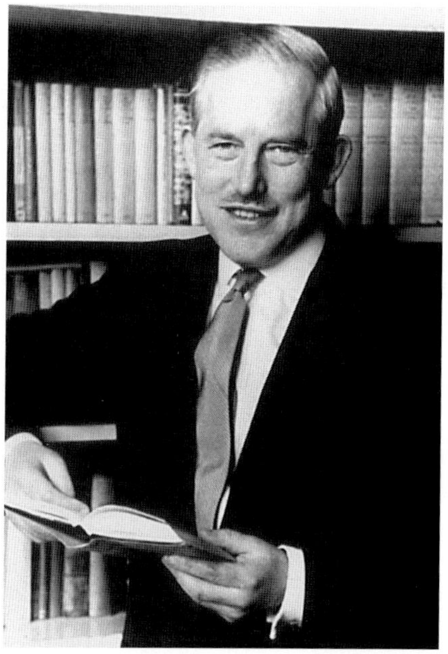

Fig. 8. Prof. O. Fitzgerald.

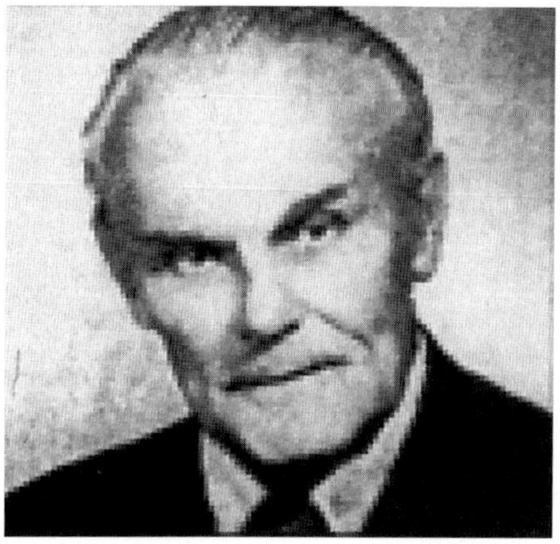

Fig. 9. Prof. K. Herfort.

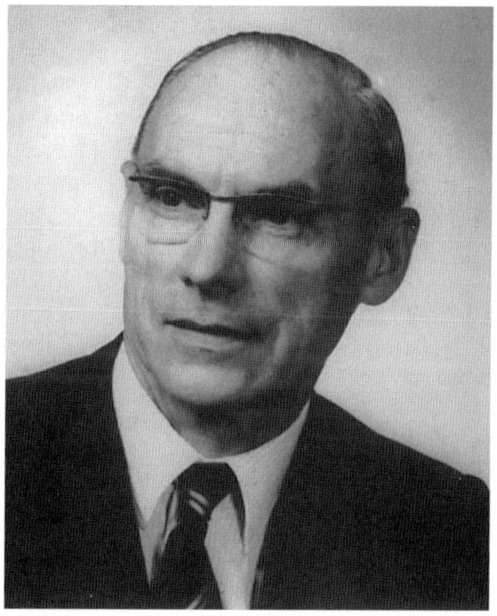

Fig. 10. Prof. H.T. Howat.

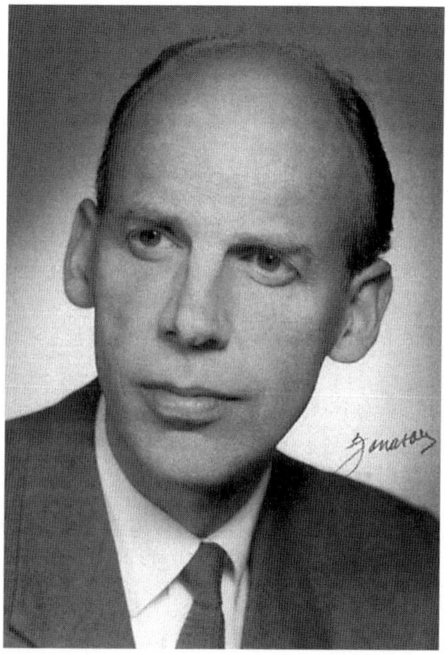

Fig. 11. Prof. Y. Edlund.

curred in a rather intense political atmosphere from the 2 to 4 July during the short 'Prague Spring'. Shortly after the end of the meeting, the Soviet Army invaded the country. So everybody who attended this meeting, including the authors, remembers those days very well. The proceedings of this symposium were published by the Czechoslovak Medical Press under the title *Progress in Pancreatology* [8]. Thirty-four papers were published, some in full length and some as abstracts. The topics were alimentary and related polypeptide hormones, pancreatic hy-

Table 3. Meetings of the EPC

	Year	Month	Place	President
1	1965	9–10 December	London, UK	H.T. Howat
2	1967	28–29 April	Marseilles, France	H. Sarles
3	1968	2–4 July	Prague, Czech Republic	K. Herfort
4	1969	26–27 September	Göttingen, Germany	W. Creutzfeldt
5	1971	16–17 April	Brussels, Belgium	J. Christophe
6	1973	24–26 May	Gothenburg, Sweden	Y. Edlund
7	1974	4–6 July	Dundee, UK	K. Wormsley
8	1975	23–25 October	Toulouse, France	A. Ribet
9	1976	14–16 October	Oslo, Norway	J. Myren
10	1977	6–8 October	Dublin, Ireland	O. Fitzgerald
11	1978	24–26 August	Zürich, Switzerland	R. Ammann
12	1979	11–13 October	Copenhagen, Denmark	H. Worning
13	1981	14–16 May	Krakow, Poland	S.J. Konturek
14	1982	30 Sept. to 2 October	Essen, Germany	H. Goebell
15	1983	29 Sept. to 1 October	Verona, Italy	L.A. Scuro
16	1984	12–14 September	Cascais, Portugal	O. Bordalo
17	1985	23–25 September	Manchester, UK	M. Case
18	1986	18–20 September	Nijmegen, The Netherlands	J.J. de Pont
19	1987	3–5 September	Marseilles, France	H. Sarles
20	1988	29–31 August	Budapest, Hungary	M. Papp
21	1989	20–23 September	Glasgow, UK	C.W. Imrie
22	1990	15–17 October	Basel, Switzerland	K. Gyr
23	1991	11–14 October	Lund, Sweden	I. Ihse
24	1992	11–14 October	Ulm, Germany	H. Beger
25	1993	20–23 October	Paris, France	C. Rozé
26	1994	7–10 September	Bologna, Italy	L. Gullo
27	1995	28 June to 1 July	Barcelona, Spain	L. Fernandez-Cruz
28[a]	1996	12–15 June	Mannheim, Germany	M.V. Singer
29	1997	9–12 July	London, UK	G.E. Mann
30	1998	10–13 June	Thessaloniki, Greece	C. Arvanitakis
31	1999	28 June to 3 July	Lüneburg, Germany	P.G. Lankisch
32	2000	28 June to 1 July	Kiel, Germany	U.R. Fölsch
33	2001	13–16 June	Toulouse, France	N. Vaysse
34[b]	2002	19–22 June	Heidelberg, Germany	M.W. Büchler
35	2003	18–22 June	Liverpool, UK	O.H. Petersen
36	2004	23–26 June	Padova, Italy	S. Pedrazzoli
37	2005	6–8 July	Graz, Austria	T. Grieshaber

[a] Joint Meeting with the IAP (C.W. Imrie).
[b] 2nd Joint Meeting with the IAP (J.P. Neoptolemos).

drolases, surgical treatment of pancreatitis and 15 free papers. Some of the presentations had the character of 'state of the art lectures' (J.E. Jorpes, V. Mutt, M.I. Grossman, H. Sarles, H.T. Howat, Y. Edlund), others presented new results, mainly in the Free Paper Session. So the symposium had a mixed character that represented the interests of the time.

The EPC from 1969 to 1980: The Transition from Symposia to Meetings and the Development of 'Internal Rules'

In the following years, with the 4th symposium in Göttingen in 1969 (W. Creutzfeldt), the 5th symposium in Brussels in 1971 (J. Christophe), and the 6th symposium in Gothenburg in 1973 (Y. Edlund), it was obvious that interest in this kind of informal meetings was growing,

Table 4. Number of participants, and submitted and accepted abstracts at the meetings of the EPC

No.	Year	Place	Partici-pants	Submitted abstracts	Accepted abstracts	Publication
1	1965	London	25	?	11	Gut
2	1967	Marseilles	75	?	34	Arch Mal Appar Dig
3	1968	Prague	119	?	37	Czechoslovak Medical Press
4	1969	Göttingen	?	?	48	Faculty print
5	1971	Brussels	139	?	64	Faculty print
6	1973	Gothenburg	145	?	90	Faculty print
7	1974	Dundee	155	?	69	Faculty print
8	1975	Toulouse	184	?	105	Faculty print
9	1976	Oslo	107	?	83	Scand J Gastroenterol
10	1977	Dublin	180	?	141	Ir J Med Sci
11	1978	Zürich	130	?	89	Gastroenterol Clin Biol
12	1979	Copenhagen	182	180	139	Dan Med Bull
13	1981	Krakow	153	140	122	Faculty print
14	1982	Essen	230	170	149	Digestion
15	1983	Verona	210	230	131	Digestion
16	1984	Cascais	158	153	123	Digestion
17	1985	Manchester	210	170	150	Digestion
18	1986	Nijmegen	208	171	151	Digestion
19	1987	Marseilles	220	175	151	Digestion
20	1988	Budapest	245	172	150	Digestion
21	1989	Glasgow	218	210	176	Digestion
22	1990	Basel	246	237	167	Digestion
23	1991	Lund	235	200	150	Digestion
24	1992	Ulm	461	221	156	Digestion
25	1993	Paris	?	?	147	Digestion
26	1994	Bologna	285	215	180	Digestion
27	1995	Barcelona	277	189	160	Digestion
28	1996	Mannheim	561	312	264	Digestion
29	1997	London	?	?	225	Digestion
30	1998	Thessaloniki	286	238	174	Digestion
31	1999	Lüneburg	372	204	150	Digestion
32	2000	Kiel	231	170	152	Digestion
33	2001	Toulouse	318	184	159	Pancreatology
32	2002	Heidelberg	525	345	331	Pancreatology
33	2003	Liverpool	315	170	170	Pancreatology
34	2004	Padova	344	239	198	Pancreatology

especially also among young researchers. This led to the decision of the Council to organize symposia of the EPC on an annual basis. In 1979, due to the growing size and the now accepted duration of 2.5 days the term 'symposium' was replaced by 'meeting'. The meeting on an annual basis, with one exception in 1980, due to interference with the World Congress of Gastroenterology in Hamburg, was continued. The EPC meeting of 1980 was postponed at the request of the President S. Konturek by 1 year.

In table 3 all meetings of the EPC from 1965 through 2005 with their Presidents are listed and in table 4 the number of participants, the submitted and accepted presentations and the organ of publication. At the 2nd meeting in Marseilles, 1967, 75 participants were counted, while at the 3rd meeting in Prague, 1968, there were 119. The number of attendants then increased steadily. At the 5th meeting in Brussels, 1971, 139 people participated and presented 64 papers. Ten years later, in 1983 (the 15th meeting in Verona), 210 researchers attended. This figure with numbers between 200 and 250 attendants interestingly has remained fairly stable until the present. It seems to represent the critical number of researchers in Europe, who are interested in the pancreas and in this kind of meeting. This figure highlights the number of all the people who work on problems of the pancreas in European hospitals and institutes. However, if we compare this with the liver and heart researchers, there are not so many. Since 1992 more than 250 attendants were registered 9 times and more than 400 3 times. The number of abstracts, which were submitted and accepted, increased from the early years (30–60) to about 180 per meeting in the1980s. This number is nearly the same as that of the attendants; this demonstrates that the active researchers come to the meetings. On average, 75% of the submitted papers are accepted for presentation. At the 1977 meeting in Dublin (President O. Fitzgerald), for the first time poster sessions were introduced. They received good acceptance, although the advantages were discussed. With an experienced older member as a moderator the sessions were well organized. The oral presentations were limited to about 25.

The years from 1970 to 1980 mark a phase of consolidation of the EPC. More and more researchers were attracted, not only across Europe, but also in the USA and other countries. A special concern was the involvement of researchers from eastern countries. Whenever possible, the Presidents of the Club helped with invitations and travel grants. Ideas were developed relatively early on how and where it might be possible to have meetings of the EPC in Eastern European countries behind the 'Iron Curtain'. The Prague Symposium in 1968 actually was the first one in Eastern Europe, Krakow (1981) and Budapest (1988) followed later.

Internal Rules

The step by step development of Internal Rules was very important in the consolidation of the Club. For many years the EPC was a rather informal association without statutes. It had no official list of members and no membership fee. A person usually was invited to the two next meetings after attending one or two prior meetings. Annual meeting attendance was open to all people actively engaged in pancreatic research. The EPC conferences from the beginning were aimed at the multidisciplinary integration of basic scientists and clinicians, i.e. medical and surgical pancreatologists and pathologists. This integration was made easier and put on a personal basis by the familiar character of the meetings. Young investigators were especially encouraged to attend the meetings. It was easy for them to get to know the leaders in the field of their research. This kind of informality led to a good number of new contacts, new cooperation, exchange of people and methodologies with other international laboratories and hospitals. It offered the clinical researchers the possibility of adopting the approach of the basic scientists to the problems of research in clinical departments and laboratories, i.e. the pathophysiology of pancreatic secretion in the diseased pancreas, the development of new tests for pancreatic function, and the research with gastrointestinal hormones in disease (for instance in hormone-producing tumors). In view of the multilinguistic European society, presentations in English, German and French were accepted in the first years, but since the early 1970s English has become the official language of the meetings.

At the 6th symposium in Gothenburg in 1973, four of the founding members left the Council, W. Creutzfeldt (Germany), A. Delcourt (Belgium), A.A. Harper (UK) and H.T. Howat (UK), and were replaced by H. Schmidt (Germany), T. Scratcherd (UK), K.G. Wormsley (UK) and H. Worning (Denmark). At the same time the term Council was replaced by Executive Council or Committee. The transition from the founders to the younger generation was possible without a break due to the fixed and written Internal Rules for the business of the Club. These had been formulated on the initiative of H. Sarles in 1973 and were accepted by a vote of the General Assembly at the 6th meeting in Gothenburg. This step was so important for the future of the EPC that the full text is given here:

'Rules of the European Pancreatic Club, 1973'

1 The association shall be called the European Pancreatic Club. Its object shall be the study of exocrine pancreatic function and disease.
2 The meetings of the Club shall be conducted in a manner to facilitate the interchange of information and promote friendship among those who have a special interest in the study of the pancreas.
3 Attendance at the meetings shall be open to all who are actively engaged in research on the pancreas. Invitations for the two forthcoming meetings will be sent to participants of the previous two meetings.
4 The business of the Club shall be conducted by an Executive Council comprising a president, the immediate past president and six committee members.
5 The president shall be elected at each meeting on the recommendation of the Council. He will preside over the Club and shall be ex officio a member of the Council for that year. The six ordinary members of the Council shall serve for a period of three meetings and are not eligible for immediate re-election. Two members will be elected at each meeting by the assembly.

Suggestions for nominations should be sent to the secretary more than two months prior to the meeting. In the case of a vacancy the Council shall nominate a substitute of the same nationality to serve for the unexpired period. The Council will designate one of its members to act as secretary and one as treasurer. Transitional rule: In 1973, 6 members will be elected, two of them will serve for one year, two for two years and two for a full three years.

6 Only registered participants of European countries are allowed to vote at the meeting.

7 The president may elect a local secretary from among members of his own country to assist him in the organisation of the next meeting.

8 The treasurer shall receive subscriptions, pay all bills and present the accounts of the Club yearly to the Executive Council and to the General Meeting.

9 The secretary shall summon all meetings of the Club and Council, shall maintain a nominal role of members and shall keep brief minutes of what passes. He shall send, not less than two months before the General Meeting to each member of the Club, a list of candidates for the various offices.

10 Meetings of the Club shall be held each year preferably in September in the country of the president. The meeting shall ordinarily last three days (Thursday, Friday and Saturday).

11 New European guests may be introduced by members to the scientific meetings of the Club. They may submit papers and take part in discussions.

12 Scientific communications shall be selected by a Committee comprising the president and two designated members of the Council. Short communications in English of two hundred and fifty words should be sent to the president some twelve weeks before the Meeting. Abstracts selected for the Meeting will be circulated if possible to all registered participants before the Meeting. Communications shall not exceed 10 min to permit ample time for discussion. The papers may be presented in any European language.

13 Members will finance their own journeys to meetings and accommodation.

14 Central funds will be built up to permit paying of fares of invited speakers. These would be associate members of the meeting. They will not have voting rights of full members but may be invited to talk to the Club because of some particular interest or development of their research.

15 The working rules of the Club shall be changed only at a business meeting by a two-thirds majority.'

Table 5. The officers of the EPC

Secretary	
1965–1973	None
1974–1976	Helmut Schmidt, Göttingen, Germany
1977–1981	Harald Goebell, Essen, Germany
1982–1985	Ulrich R. Foelsch, Göttingen and Kiel, Germany
1986–1992	Manfred V. Singer, Essen and Mannheim, Germany
1993–1997	Jan. J. Jansen, Nijmegen, The Netherlands
1998–2002	John P. Neoptolemos, Liverpool, UK
2003 up to the present	Markus Lerch, Greifswald, Germany
Treasurer	
1965–1974	None
1975	Tim Scratcherd, Newcastle, UK
1976–1977	Helge Worning, Copenhagen, Denmark
1978–1989	Rudolf Ammann, Zürich, Switzerland
1990–1992	Harald Goebell, Essen, Germany
1993–1996	Klaus Gyr, Basel, Switzerland
1997 up to the present	Christoph Beglinger, Basel, Switzerland

The introduction of these rules stabilized the EPC in the forthcoming years. The six council members were all from different countries with a limited term of 3 years, with an equal representation of basic and clinical investigators. The elected President was responsible for organizing the meetings in his country. The appointment of a General Secretary and of a Treasurer were also important steps. Table 5 lists the officers of the EPC from 1974 to 2003. The terms of the officers changed somewhat individually, but on average it was 5 years, or 2 terms for the treasurer.

The introduction of a Selection Committee for the submitted papers was also new. From 1974 to 1975 it was the President plus 2 members, from 1976 to 1978 the President plus 3 members and from 1979 to1988 the President plus 4 members. In 1989 the Selection Committee was increased to 8 members, 4 for basic and 4 for clinical sciences, serving for 2 years. Because of the requirement that the individual countries should be represented and at the same time also the need that those selected would be competent, the selection process had to be carried out with great sensitivity.

With the new rules there was a transition period from the Council of the founders to an Elected Committee, which lasted from 1973 to 1976. Yngve Edlund, Karel Herfort, Henri Sarles and Jean Christophe left the Council in 1975. They were replaced by Stanislaw J. Konturek (Poland), Rudolf Ammann (Switzerland) and André Ri-

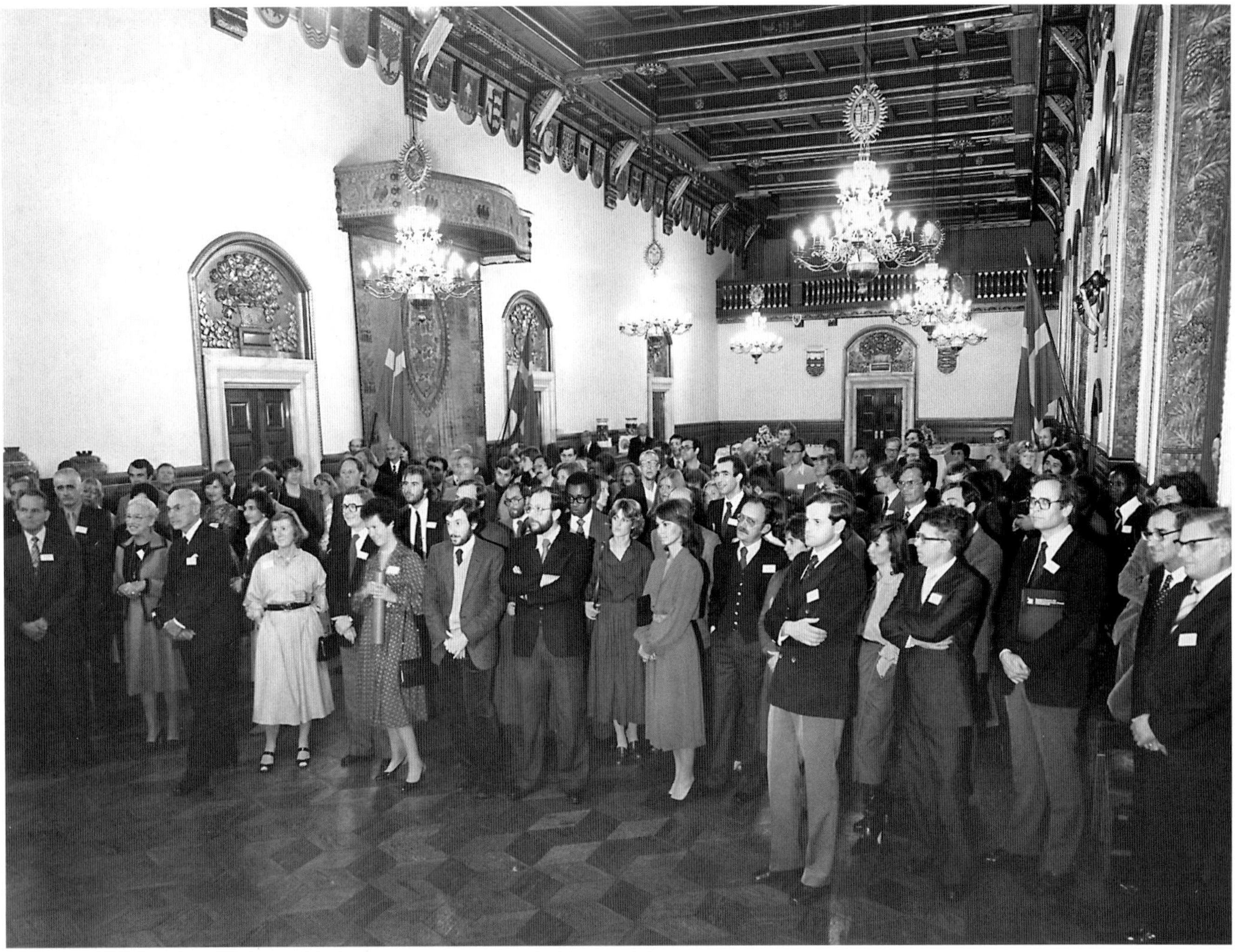

Fig. 12. 12th Symposium EPC – Copenhagen, October 11–13, 1979. President: Helge Worning. Welcome reception.

bet (France). Helmut Schmidt (Germany) became the first Secretary of the Club in 1974. He served until 1976. Rudolf Ammann came into office as Treasurer after a short transition period (Tim Scratcherd in 1975, Helge Worning in 1976/1977) in 1978 and served in this function until 1989 (table 5).

Social Functions of the Club

From the very beginning it was felt to be very important for the exchange between basic and clinical scientists and the development of friendships across borders to have social events during the EPC meetings emphasizing the familiar character of the Club. So a welcome evening (fig. 12) and a gala banquet (fig. 13) usually with dancing became integrated parts of the meetings. Other cultural events like visits to museums and also invitations to the homes of the local scientists were highly appreciated. An important role was always played by the partners of the members and also by a good ladies program. There is no doubt that all this contributed to significant and often long-lasting friendships and collaborations.

Figure 14 gives a view of the lecture hall during the EPC meeting in Zürich in 1978.

The EPC from 1980 to 1990 and the Relation to Other Scientific Societies

On the basis of the new rules of 1973 the EPC developed steadily with increasing acceptance. This is mirrored by an increasing number of participants to an average of 200 at each meeting. The number of abstracts

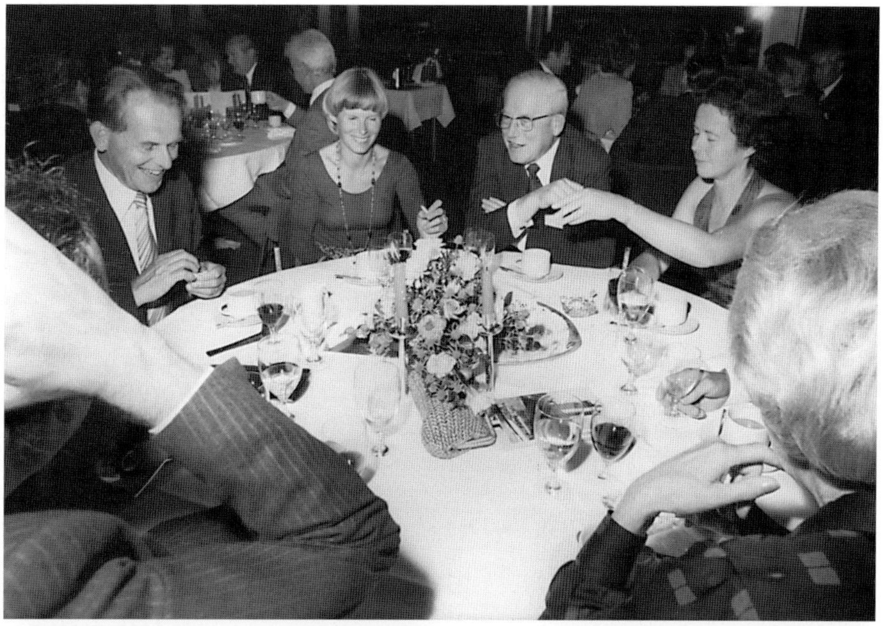

Fig. 13. 11th Symposium EPC – Zürich, 1978. Gala dinner. From left to right: Rudolf Ammann (President), Rosemarie Goebell, Oliver Fitzgerald, and Marianne Ammann.

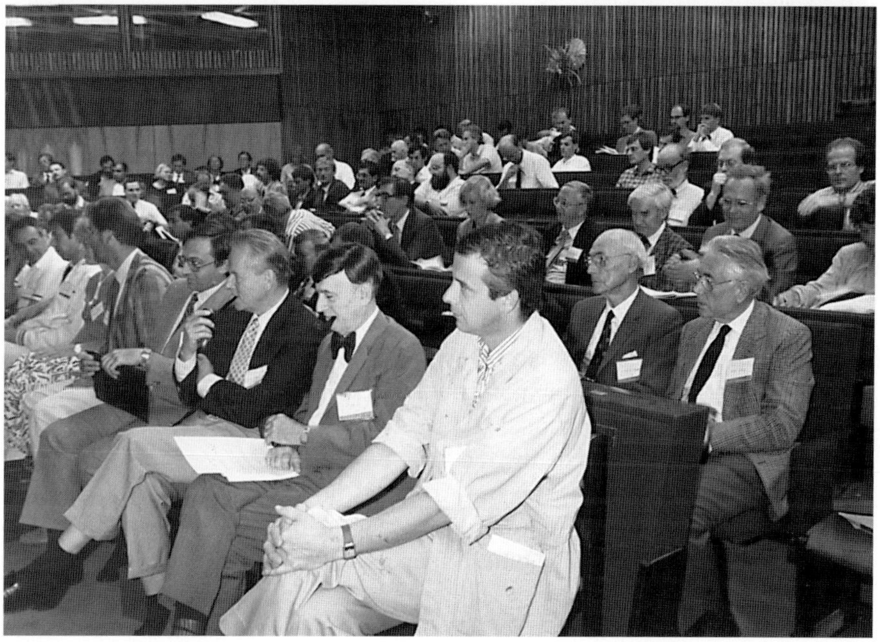

Fig. 14. 11th Symposium EPC – Zürich, 1978. President: R. Ammann. Rudolf Ammann (row 1: 3rd person, right to left), D.A. Dreiling (row 1: 2nd person, right to left), H. Sarles (row 2: 1st person, right), H.T. Howat (row 2: 2nd person, right to left), and H. Goebell (row 3: 2nd person, right to left).

submitted oscillated between 150 and 350, of which around 150 were accepted (table 4).

An important issue was the publication of the abstracts of the accepted papers. In the years from 1969 to 1981 they were presented to the members during the meetings as faculty prints or in some years in national journals (table 4). In 1982 the Club reached an agreement with Karger Publishers with the help of W. Creutzfeldt who was at that time Editor-in-Chief of *Digestion*. The affiliation with *Digestion* for the printing of the abstracts lasted 19 years until 2000 (32nd meeting in Kiel). After intense discussions it was then decided to change to the journal *Pancreatology*, also published by Karger. This was done for the first time at the Toulouse meeting in 2001. *Pancreatology* from that date has been the official journal of the EPC and of the International Association of Pancreatology (IAP) and of five other national pancreatic societies. Here it should be mentioned that the foun-

Table 6. Origin of accepted and printed abstracts at the meetings of the EPC

	1971–1980	1981–1990	1991–2000	2001–2004	Total
Austria	4	–	5	6	15
Belgium	48	30	11	9	98
Denmark	31	33	23	4	91
Finland	–	8	7	24	39
France	166	216	133	60	575
Germany	156	386	460	229	1,231
UK	126	187	148	110	571
Hungary	12	53	41	69	175
Ireland	14	10	2	2	28
Italy	51	139	228	49	467
The Netherlands	18	75	31	15	139
Norway	7	–	–	2	9
Poland	10	32	53	94	189
Portugal	7	–	–	–	7
Spain	8	17	123	43	191
Sweden	26	70	121	35	252
Switzerland	12	50	74	12	160
USA/Canada	31	48	60	53	352
Other countries outside central Europe (i.e. Eastern Europe, Asia, South America), sporadically					248
Total					4,837

dation of the EPC in 1965 had an enormous positive influence on the development of pancreatology in the European countries as is documented by the foundation of many small regional 'clubs', making the EPC, so to speak, their 'mother'. The international acceptance of the EPC is reflected by the number of abstracts not only from European countries but also from the Americas and Asia. Table 6 lists the countries according to their contribution to the scientific sessions. The bulk of papers came from Germany, France, UK and Italy. Other European countries with a considerable number of contributions were Belgium, Denmark, The Netherlands, Hungary, Poland, Spain, Sweden and Switzerland. We always had guests from the USA. They contributed 352 original papers to the meetings of the EPC.

In the years from 1980 to 1990 one of the most important topics of discussion in the Executive Committee and in the General Assembly was the relationship to other supranational societies with an interest in pancreatology. As early as 1974 David A. Dreiling, New York, N.Y. tried to persuade the EPC to found a World Pancreatic Society, mainly including the EPC, the American Pancreatic Association (APA) and the American Pancreatic Club. This proposal was unanimously declined. The main arguments were that young members cannot travel all over the world to meetings and the informal and stimulating character of the EPC meetings would be lost.

In 1983 a new initiative for the foundation of a bigger worldwide acting society, the International Association of Pancreatology (IAP), was started by Orlando Bordalo from Portugal, a pupil of D.A. Dreiling. It was supported by colleagues from Italy, Portugal, South America, some from the USA but not many from other European countries. The proposal was to have meetings along with the World Congress of Gastroenterology and from time to time together with the EPC or the APA or the Japanese Pancreatic Association. After intense discussions at the EPC the unanimous opinion was not to support the foundation of this new society. Nevertheless, the IAP was founded in Cascais in 1984. They had a first but separate meeting without the participation of the EPC, which had its 16th meeting in the same week also in Cascais under the presidency of O. Bordalo. The situation was very delicate.

Fortunately matters improved in the following years. The IAP developed separately, especially under US influence. As a matter of fact, many European researchers are now members of both societies. The IAP meets every 4 years. The EPC has since delegated a member to the executive council of the IAP.

In 1996 the first joint meeting of the EPC (President Manfred V. Singer) and the IAP (President Clem W. Imrie) took place in Mannheim. A second joint meeting was held in Heidelberg 2002 with Markus W. Büchler as President of the EPC and John P. Neoptolemos as President of the IAP. Both meetings had a high standard and attracted many participants; the IAP side mainly consisted of surgeons. The next joint meeting of the EPC with the IAP will take place in Lodz, Poland, in 2008 under the EPC presidency of Eva Malecka-Panas and the IAP presidency of Markus Lerch.

At the 20th EPC meeting in Budapest in 1988 David A. Dreiling made another plea to the EPC and the IAP to form one single club. But this was again refused.

At the 17th meeting of the EPC in Manchester in 1985 and under the presidency of Maynard Case, the founding member Henry T. Howat gave an Anniversary Dinner Talk at the banquet on the occasion of the 20th anniversary of the foundation of the EPC. He reflected on the 20 years of a successful development of a well-renowned scientific society.

The Years 1990–1992 and the Transition of the EPC to an Official Society with New Statutes

In the years 1989 and 1990 the Association des Sociétés Nationales Européennes et Méditerranéennes de Gastroentérologie (ASNEMGE) under the presidency of A. Torsoli, Italy, and the Secretary General R.H. Dowling, UK, started an initiative to create a United European Gastroenterology Week (UEGW). The representatives of seven European (not national) societies, among them the EPC, were invited to join this initiative. The preliminary meeting took place in Rome on February 10, 1990 and the founding session in L'Aquila on April 28, 1990. The President of the EPC Klaus Gyr attended the meeting in L'Aquila. He returned with a very positive attitude to the new idea of the UEGW. In fact a united meeting of several small societies in Europe, also as a counterpart to the Digestive Disease Week in the USA, seemed to be attractive for gastroenterologists in Europe, especially in the Eastern countries.

The issue of the UEGW and of its organization UEGF (United European Gastroenterology Federation) was discussed extensively by the Executive Committee of the EPC at the 22nd meeting in Basel with Klaus Gyr as President.

There was consent that: '(1) The meetings of the EPC will continue on an annual basis. In general the meeting will last two and a half days as has been the case before. The EPC wants to keep its own identity and to continue to be a club where basic and clinical scientists can meet in a familiar atmosphere to discuss science and to create new and continue old friendships. (2) The Council of the EPC expresses its general support of the ASNEMGE and (3) the EPC is prepared to organize the pancreatic session of the UEGF during the so-called United European Gastroenterology Week (UEGW)' (from the protocol of the session of the Executive Council of the EPC, Basel, 1990). K. Gyr and M.V. Singer were asked to act as delegates of the EPC to the UEGF/ASNEMGE.

It was also discussed that it was necessary to work out new statutes for the EPC (on the basis of the 1973 rules) to meet the criteria of a modern scientific society. A commission for statutes was inaugurated. The following members were designated: Ingmar Ihse (President 1991), Manfred V. Singer (Secretary), Harald Goebell (Treasurer), Clem W. Imrie (Past President 1989), Maynard Case (Past President 1985) and Nicole Vaysse (Toulouse). A time schedule was recommended with the presentation of a first draft to the Executive Committee in the course of 1991 and to the General Assembly at the meeting in Lund in 1991. The plan for the final vote on the new statutes was to be taken by the General Assembly at the meeting in Ulm in 1992.

In 1991 M.V. Singer prepared a draft of the statutes which was distributed among the members of the special committee and discussed at the regular meeting of the official boards in Lund. M.V. Singer was asked to work out, on the basis of the first draft, a final version with the statute committee, to present this version to all registered members of the Club, and to ask for their comments and proposals. This big action indeed happened during 1992 and the Secretary presented a final version of the statutes to the General Assembly in Ulm after approval by the Council. Interestingly there was again a lively discussion about the necessity of the new statutes, which demonstrated how much the members treasured the informality of the Club. But finally everybody was convinced and the new statutes were approved by an almost unanimous vote (three votes against, one withheld).

So after 3 years of really democratic work the Club had new statutes. After this vote the General Assembly decided on the proposals of the Council for the different offices, the Presidents and places of the forthcoming meetings up to 1996, the Secretary of the Club for the next 5 years (Jan Jansen, Nijmegen), the new Treasurer (Klaus Gyr), the Council with 6 members and the Abstract Selection Committee (four basic and four clinical scientists). As delegate of the EPC to the IAP C. Beglinger (Switzerland) was elected and as delegates to the UEGF K. Gyr and M.V. Singer. At the end of the Ulm Meeting the President Hans G. Beger thanked Manfred V. Singer for his immense dedication to the creation of the new statutes. Without his commitment the transition of the EPC to an official society would not have occurred in such a smooth manner.

The new statutes of 1992 were formed on the basis of the rules of the EPC from 1973. In five articles name, purpose and status (1), membership (2), powers (3), meetings (4) and change of statutes (5) were defined. Membership required a membership fee, which is set by the General Assembly on the proposal of the Council. The composition of the Executive Council was not changed (President, Secretary, Treasurer and six councillors and the Past President). The election of all officers now became the task of the General Assembly on the proposal of the Council. It was ascertained that the meetings will be held annually with a duration of 2.5 days. Members of the Selection Committee for the scientific communications are the President ex officio and four members for basic and four for clinical sciences. These members are elected by the General Assembly for 2 years on the proposal of the Council. A registration fee in addition to the membership fee is payable at the meetings. The new statutes were accepted unanimously and did not change the essential character of the meetings.

From this day forward the EPC was also represented on the boards of the UEGF actively organizing half a pancreas day at the UEGW. The first such meeting was held in Athens in1993.

The EPC from 1993 to 2005

In the years after the introduction of the new statutes the Club developed steadily. In the 1990s the number of participants usually was between 200 and 250 with many new young researchers. In 1996 the first joint meeting of the EPC and AIP took place in Mannheim (President M.V. Singer). The second joint meeting was organized in Heidelberg 2002 by the Presidents M.W. Büchler and J.P. Neoptolemos. In 1997 it was decided that the executive council should meet twice yearly at the EPC meeting and in connection with the UEGW to deal with all issues properly. The financial situation of the Club was good. Therefore, it started to create an EPC scholarship for annual travel grants to young investigators. In 2004, for instance, a total of 36 travel awards and 2 best abstract prizes were awarded. The travel awards were given to 8 basic scientists, to 18 scientists involved in experimental pathophysiological work and to 10 scientists doing pure clinical work. The best abstract prizes were given to 1 scientist for basic and 1 for clinical work.

The Young Researchers Corner, a new category of scientific information, was introduced by President Claude Rozé for the first time at the 25th meeting in Paris in 1993. Its purpose was the postgraduate training of members in research techniques. So in Paris 'cultured cells, receptors, cell pathing and calcium imaging' were discussed. This new form of information is now regularly organized at each meeting with much success (for more details see part 2 of this article).

A new category of activities at the EPC was opened in 1995 at the 27th meeting in Barcelona with the inauguration of cooperative studies among members. A European Study Group of Pancreatic Cancer (ESPAC) held the first meeting in Barcelona under the chairmanship of H.G. Beger, J.P. Neoptolemos, and M.W. Büchler. The group now meets regularly at the EPC. At present it runs three different studies (for details see part 2 of this article). A European register for Hereditary Pancreatitis and Familial Pancreatic Cancer was opened at the 33rd meeting in Toulouse in 2001. Since 2001 the topic of hereditary diseases of the pancreas is run under the title EUROPAC (European Registry of Hereditary Pancreatitis and Familial Pancreatic Cancer).

A new attractive logo was developed by Thomas Griesbacher and accepted in 2000 in Kiel. In 2001 the EPC organized its own website: www.e-p-c.org. In 1999 a News Letter was published for the first time. Number 6 came out in 2004. The Secretary of the Club is the editor. The EPC created an award medal for outstanding work for the Club and for pancreatology. In 2001 it was presented in Toulouse to Rudolf Ammann and Hans G. Beger. Also in 2001 the journal *Pancreatology* was chosen for the publication of abstracts and as their official organ at the suggestion of Markus Lerch and with an unanimous Council vote. A triple membership was offered to the members of the EPC, the IAP and the National Pancreatic Associations in Europe combined with automatic subscription to *Pancreatology*. In 2003 the EPC had 230 registered members. The vast majority has taken advantage of the triple membership.

Revision of the Statutes from 1992 in the Year 2001

Nevertheless, having served as a stable basis for the work of the EPC it was felt that some revision of the statutes was needed to adopt details to meet the requirements, although for the authors of this paper these requirements are not quite clear. More details in a statute are not necessarily better. In the year 2000 the Executive Council worked on this problem and in Toulouse 2001 the revised statutes were accepted by the Council and the General Assembly. Compared to the statutes of 1992 they were more detailed and precise on some issues. They now have 11 articles instead of 5: Article I: Name, Article II: Duration and Dissolution, Article III: Aims, Article IV: Membership, Article V: General Assembly, Article VI: Council, Article VII: Responsibilities of the Council, Article VIII: Quorum and Voting of the Council, Article IX: Sub-Committees, Article X: Organisation of the EPC Meeting, and Article XI: Change of Statutes. The full text of the 2001 statutes is available at the EPC website [10].

The EPC is now registered in Switzerland as an international association (Article I). The aims are much more detailed (Article III): '(A) To promote communication between basic and clinical scientists in Europe interested in the pancreas and its disorders; (B) to promote and organise an annual scientific meeting devoted to all aspects of the pancreas; (C) to promote scientific, epidemiological and clinical research into pancreatic function and into the prevention, diagnosis and therapy of pancreatic diseases. Preference will be given to co-operative projects; (D) to establish scholarships and promote postgraduate education and training; (E) to support other meetings concerning the pancreas organised by members of the EPC; (F) to disseminate information about EPC activities, and publish such educational matter as the EPC council may consider desirable.' This new definition of the aims now covered issues such as postgraduate training, cooperative studies like ESPAC and EUROPAC, and involvement in the organization of the UEGW meeting. Article V defines the role of the General Assembly, which was not the case in the statutes of 1992. The General Assembly is now characterized as being the 'highest organ of the EPC'. It decides on the proposals of the Executive Council, i.e. elections, accounts, fees, alteration of the constitution, and cooperation with other societies. A quorum is introduced with the presence of at least 30% of the members participating at the annual meeting. Voting by proxy in writing is also permitted. A single majority in votes is needed with the exception of alterations of the constitution which require a two-third majority. In Article V the Council is defined. The members are now the President, the President Elect (new), the Past President, the Secretary, the Treasurer and six Councillors from different European countries, three basic and three clinical scientists. The latter serve for 3 years, the Secretary cannot be re elected whereas the Treasurer my be reelected.

It is also new that the Presidents and the countries for the forthcoming meetings must be decided on by the General Assembly 'strictly' 4 years in advance after nomination by the Council. In Article VII concerning the responsibilities of the Council, it is new that it can delegate responsibilities to subcommittees or working parties as appropriate.

The present constitution of the EPC represents a stable and reliable base for the future. One thing must be pointed out at the end of this discourse about the history of the EPC: In the headline of the statutes it says: 'Statutes, European Pancreatic Club, Founded in 1962'. The latter is definitely wrong, as we have shown in our article. The EPC was founded in 1965 and not in 1962 (will be corrected as assured by the ECP Secretary).

The manuscript is based on the nearly complete set of programs, abstract books, drafts and final versions of the statutes, votes, minutes of the sessions of the Committee and General Assembly and many personal contacts. The material is now stored in the newly founded Archive of the European Club, which will presumably be deposited in the library of the University of Zürich, Switzerland. Until that date it is stored with Prof. Goebell, Essen [9].

Acknowledgments

We wish to thank all colleagues who helped gather all the information needed. We also thank Mrs. Rita Shinkle for checking the linguistic quality of the manuscript and Professor Maynard Case and Professor Markus Lerch for their critical and excellent remarks which improved the manuscript enormously.

References

1 Howard JM, Hess W: History of the Pancreas: Mysteries of a Hidden Organ. New York, Kluwer Academic/Plenum Publishers, 2002.
2 Satake K, Takeuchi T: Brief history of the Japan Pancreas Society. Pancreas 1998;16:432–433.
3 Frey CF, Schiller WJ: Introduction to the history of the pancreas club. J Gastrointest Surg 2004;8(suppl):S1–S14.
4 de Reuck AVS, Cameron MP: Ciba Foundation Symposium on the Exocrine Pancreas: Normal and Abnormal Functions. London, Churchill, 1962.
5 Sarles H: Pancreatitis. Symposium Marseille, April 25–26, 1963. Bibliotheca Gastroenterologica. Basel, Karger, 1965, No 7.
6 Howat HT: European Pancreatic Club. Gut 1966;7:298–302.
7 Sarles H : Deuxième Colloque Européen du Pancréas, 28 et 29 avril 1967, Marseille. Arch Fr Mal Appar Dig 1967;56:993–1006.
8 Fric P, Malis F, Ronsky R: Progress in Pancreatology. Proceedings of the Third Symposium of the European Pancreatic Club, Prague 2nd–4th July 1968. Prague, Czechoslovak Medical Press, 1968.
9 Minutes of the Meetings of the Council of the European Pancreatic Club 1976 to 2003. c/o Prof. Dr. Goebell, Schinkelstr. 34, DE–45138 Essen, Germany.
10 Statutes of the European Pancreatic Club revised 2001, available at the website www.e-p-c.org.

Part 2

Pancreatology

Pancreatology 2005;5(suppl 1):16–34
DOI: 10.1159/000086211

Published online: June 6, 2005

History of the European Pancreatic Club: The First 40 Years 1965–2005

The Scientific Profile of the European Pancreatic Club and What Stood the Test of Time

Harald Goebell[a] Rudolf Ammann[b] Werner Creutzfeldt[c]

[a]University of Essen, Essen, Germany; [b]University of Zurich, Zurich, Switzerland; [c]University of Göttingen, Göttingen, Germany

Abstract

The invited lectures, the symposia and panels and the printed abstracts of the meetings are the basis for analysis of the development of pancreatic research over the 40 years from 1965 to 2005. 245 invited lectures and 59 symposia, panels and round tables presented and discussed the latest state of the art at the meetings of the European Pancreatic Club (EPC). We analyze in detail the contributions to physiology and biochemistry of the pancreas, the neurohormonal control of pancreatic secretion, cell biology, stimulus-secretion coupling, and cell receptors. The research on the endocrine-exocrine relationship, nutrition and the pancreas, experimental and clinical acute and chronic pancreatitis, function tests and imaging of the pancreas, pancreatic development and growth, experimental and clinical pancreatic carcinoma, genetics and inherited pancreatic diseases over the years are listed in special sections and discussed. At the center of the EPC meetings there are scientific sessions with either oral or poster presentations. From 1971 to 2004, 4,837 contributions were accepted and printed as abstracts. In the first 30 years papers on basic research usually amounted to around 30–40%, on pathophysiology also 20–40% and the rest were on clinical work. In the years since 1993 the basic contributions became less with 20% and even only 10% of all papers in the last years. Abstracts from pathophysiology and pathology increased in the 1990s, mainly with work on pancreatic carcinoma. Papers on clinical topics also rose to 40–50% of all in the years since 1998. The interest in clinical topics shifted over the years. Chronic pancreatitis was the main topic in the 1970s; in the 1980s until 2000, acute pancreatitis gained more interest, and pancreatic cancer is now an attractive field of study due to new methods of research with cancer cell lines and genetic models. Since 1993 a Young Researchers Corner with international experts is offered at the meetings of the EPC, the programs are analyzed. In the last section the question of 'what stood the test of time?' is asked as reflected in 40 years of meetings of the EPC. Topics are physiology, biochemistry and cell biology in relation to the pancreas, pathogenesis of acute and chronic pancreatitis, methods of diagnosis, treatment of pancreatitis and of carcinoma.

The Scientific Profile of the European Pancreatic Club

The founders of the European Pancreatic Club (EPC) intended to create a forum, where European scientists with an interest in the pancreas could meet and discuss

KARGER

Fax +41 61 306 12 34
E-Mail karger@karger.ch
www.karger.com

© 2005 S. Karger AG, Basel, IAP and EPC
1424–3903/05/0057–0016$22.00/0

Accessible online at:
www.karger.com/pan

Prof. emeritus Dr. Harald Goebell
Department of Gastroenterology and Hepatology
University of Essen, Universitätsklinikum, Hufelandstrasse 55
DE–45122 Essen (Germany)
Tel. +49 201 263355, Fax +49 201 2667393, E-Mail harald.goebell@uni-essen.de

Table 1. Number of invited lectures at the meetings of the EPC from 1968 to 2004 and nationality of the lecturers

Number of invited lectures

1968	1969	1971	1973	1974	1975	1976	1977	1978	1979	1981	1982
Prague	Göttingen	Brussels	Gothenburg	Dundee	Toulouse	Oslo	Dublin	Zürich	Copenhagen	Krakow	Essen
12	none	3	7	1	3	2	2	2	2	3	2
1983	1984	1985	1986	1987	1988	1989	1990	1991	1992	1993	1994
Verona	Cascais	Manchester	Nijmegen	Marseilles	Budapest	Glasgow	Basel	Lund	Ulm	Paris	Bologna
2	9	12	2	none	11	9	9	3	11	3	10
1995	1996	1997	1998	1999	2000	2001	2002	2003	2004		
Barcelona	Mannheim	London	Thessaloniki	Lüneburg	Kiel	Toulouse	Heidelberg	Liverpool	Padova		
none	23	18	12	26	15	14	6	4	7		

Nationality of invited lecturers

Germany	67	France	25	Belgium	8	Netherlands	4	Norway	3
UK	50	Italy	11	Switzerland	5	Spain	4	Israel, Poland, Austria,	
USA	38	Sweden	10	Denmark	4	Japan	3	Greece, Portugal, Hungary	1 each

Titles, lecturers and the symposia are listed in tables 2–13. We apologize for any omissions that might have occurred.

Table 2. Names of invited scientists to give lectures in their field of research

1968	Prague	Jorpes S, Mutt S, Morley UK, Anastasi I, Harper UK, Morris UK, Erspamer I, Howat UK, J.C. Sarles F, Smith UK, Edlund S, Arrigas E, Wagner D
1969	Göttingen	None
1971	Brussels	Jamieson USA, Schramm ISR, Malaisse B
1973	Gothenburg	Case UK, Christophe B, Creutzfeldt D, Worning DK, Howat UK, Schmidt D, H. Sarles F
1974	Dundee	Lagerlöf S
1975	Toulouse	Scratcherd UK, Meldolesi I, H. Sarles F
1976	Oslo	Petersen N, Creutzfeldt D
1977	Dublin	H. Sarles F, Konturek PL
1978	Zürich	Christophe B, Seifert D
1979	Copenhagen	Bloom UK, Wormsley UK
1981	Krakow	Schaffalitzky de Muckadell DK, Creutzfeldt D, Wormsley UK
1982	Essen	Kern D, Malaisse D
1983	Verona	Solcia I, DiMagno USA
1984	Cascais	Case UK, Bockmann USA, Creutzfeldt D, Go USA, H. Sarles F, Lees UK, Goebell D, Domschke D, Joyeux F
1985	Manchester	Scheele USA, Kern D, Bockmann USA, Foulis UK, Braganza UK, Noronha P, Vaysse F, Dormer UK, Lees UK, Williamson UK, Klapdor D, Singer D
1986	Nijmegen	McMaster UK, Geuze NL
1987	Marseilles	None
1988	Budapest	Ammann CH, Dreiling USA, Howat UK, H. Sarles F, Singer D, Vaysse F, Case UK, Goebell D, Gullo I, Imrie UK, Nagy HU
1989	Glasgow	Foulis UK, Freeney USA, Garber UK, Henriksen DK, Laugier F, Carter UK, Hermon-Taylor UK, Vaysse F, Adler D
1990	Basel	Rommens CAN, Dobelbower USA, Dagorn F, Adler D, Ensinck USA, Alberti UK, Gerzof USA, Rösch D, Wynick UK
1991	Lund	Ammann CH, Mitelman S, Braganza UK
1992	Ulm	Petersen UK, Creutzfeldt D, Case UK, Vaysse F, Korc CAN, Schmiegel D, Trede D, Klöppel D, Steer USA, Christophe B, Neoptolemos UK
1993	Paris	Lamberts NL, Williams USA, Halliwell UK
1994	Bologna	H. Sarles F, Mann UK, Frey USA, Jensen USA, Singer D, LaVecchia I, Sutherland USA, Erlansson S, Mastella I
1995	Barcelona	None
1996	Mannheim	Gyr CH, Schölmerich D, Wigmore UK, Laubenberger D, Chalmers UK, Reske D, Nagoya JAP, Weber USA, Solomon USA, Bockman USA, Ammann CH, Schmiegel D, Lemoine UK, Urrutia USA, McKay UK, Larssonn S, Pollak CAN, Moore CAN, Hoolingsworth USA, Bramhall UK, Fink D, Kimura JAP, Trede D
1997	London	Müller-Esterl D, Griesbacher A, Lerch D, Klöppel D, Gearing UK, Lemoine UK, Sies D, Vina E, Moncada UK, Eizirik B, Beglinger CH, Laugier F, Petersen UK, Ashcroft UK, Gray UK, Kanno JAP, Saklatvala UK, Goris NL
1998	Thessaloniki	Mann UK, Calvo I, Cremer B, Layer D, Fölsch D, Nousia-Arvanitakis GR, Whitcomb USA, Lankisch D, Dagorn F, Vaysse F, Erlansson S, Petersen UK
1999	Lüneburg	Williams USA, Muallem USA, Miller USA, Tsunoda USA, Buscail F, Lerch D, Saluja USA, Ullrich 2nd USA, Borgström S, McMahon UK, McKay UK, Rathmann D, Scolapio USA, Merkrod D, Singer D, Tiemann D, Mössner D, Adler D, Cohn USA, Creutzfeldt D, Gudjonsson N, Johnson UK, Kalthoff D, Gansauge D, Friess D, Löhr D
2000	Kiel	Rathmann D, Moreau USA, Lemoine UK, Riemann D, Weber D, Buscail F, Klöppel D, Schmid D, Real E, Scarpa I, Wagner D, Kalthoff D, Pinzani I, Wison A, Sjöholm S
2001	Toulouse	Gullo I, Löhr D, Buscail F, Chen F, Witt D, Hammel F, Neoptolemos UK, Urrutia USA, Serup DK, Glasbrenner D, Layer D, Jovanna F, Van Laethem B, Escourrou F
2002	Heidelberg	Argent UK, Schmid D, Vollmar D, DiMagno USA, Obertop NL, Schmidt D
2003	Liverpool	Urrutia USA, Whitcomb USA, Muallem USA, Büchler D
2004	Padova	Kalthoff D, Gaudernack N, Fernandez-Cruz E, Bachem D, Büchler D, Wyke UK, Friess D

S = Sweden; UK = United Kingdom; I = Italy; F = France; E = Spain; D = Germany; B = Belgium; PL = Poland; USA = United States of America; ISR = Israel; P = Portugal; NL = The Netherlands; CH = Switzerland; HU = Hungary; CAN = Canada; JAP = Japan; A = Austria; GR = Greece; N = Norway.

their mutual problems and questions from different angles: anatomy, physiology, biochemistry, internal medicine and surgery. This goal was reflected by the professions of the 9 founders: 1 physiologist (A.A. Harper), 1 biochemist (J. Christophe), 2 surgeons (A. Delcourt, Y. Edlund) and 5 physicians (W. Creutzfeldt, O. Fitzgerald, K. Herfort, H.T. Howat, H. Sarles), specialized in gastroenterology. Acute pancreatitis, chronic pancreatitis and cancer of the pancreas are entities with many facets and interrelationships. The meetings have shown that clinicians learn from basic sciences by adopting their methods and applying them to the study of diseases experimentally and clinically. For clinicians the problems of conservative and surgical treatment are essential issues. The correct diagnosis leads the way to adequate treatment. Originally, the diagnosis was only based on clinical symptoms. Thereafter, biochemical and physiological methods have contributed much to a correct diagnosis, for instance by the function tests for the pancreas. Imaging of the pancreas gained increasing importance over the years, starting with angiography, scintigraphy, ultrasonography and endoscopic retrograde pancreatography (ERP) with imaging of the ducts. Now the progress lies in computerized tomography and magnetic resonance imaging, not only of the parenchyme but with contrast also of the ducts. Endoscopic ultrasound must also be mentioned.

We will follow these lines over the years as they are reflected in the meetings. We will use the invited and state-of-the-art lectures for analysis, because they demonstrate what was considered to be important at the time. The topics of symposia and panels give an additional view. We will also analyze the papers which were submitted over the years for presentation in the scientific sessions either orally or as posters.

A short study of the European pancreatic research in the EPC was presented by Andren-Sandberg and Johnson [1] at the 30th EPC meeting in 1998.

Invited Lectures and Symposia

It is a privilege of the President of an EPC meeting to invite scientists for lectures. A total of 245 of those lectures were given at the meetings from 1968 to 2004 (tables 1 and 2).

These lectures presented as state-of-the-art or key note lectures should outline the frontier in a certain field of research. In the years from 1971 to 1983, only 2–3 key lectures were given at each meeting. In 1984 for the first time more scientists were invited (n = 9). This tendency increased in the following years with an average of 10 invited lecturers. From 1996 on, it increased even further: in 1996 n = 23, in 1997 n = 18, in 1998 n = 12, in 1999 n = 26, in 2000 n = 15, and in 2001 n = 14. The reason for this inflation of invited lectures is possibly the opening of the EPC meetings to more attendants, also from outside of Europe, especially the joint meetings of the EPC with the IAP in Mannheim 1996 and in Heidelberg 2002. From 2002 on, the number of additional lectures came down again to 4–7.

The symposia, panel discussions and round tables were another instrument to keep the attendants up to date. Table 3 summarizes these events together with the respective chairmen. A total of 59 were organized between 1968 and 2004, on average 1 or 2 at each meeting. From 2002 on, a certain inflation can be observed. So in Heidelberg in 2002, eight symposia took place, in Liverpool five plus a whole day on basic science and in Padua 2004 it still was four. The analysis of the symposia and the lectures are integrated in the following sections.

Physiology and Biochemistry of the Pancreas (tables 4 and 5)

In the first meetings the structure and functional aspects of the gastrointestinal hormones were of outstanding interest. In Prague in 1968, the pioneers in the field presented their data on secretin (J.E. Jorpes), cholecystokinin-pancreozymin (V. Mutt, A.A. Harper), gastrin (J.S. Morley), and cerulein (A. Anastasi). The function of the hormones in the regulation of pancreatic secretion from there on has been a constant topic over the years, especially the fascinating interplay with the nerval regulation.

In 1975, a whole working session with K.G. Wormsley and 9 speakers dealt with 'Regulation and Adaptation of Pancreatic Secretion', and another symposium under the moderation of S.J. Konturek and 8 speakers with 'Gastrointestinal Hormones and Related Peptides'.

'Intestinal Hormones and the Exocrine Pancreas' was the title of a summarizing lecture by O. Schaffalitzky de Muckadell in 1981. Lectures on the neurohormonal regulation of secretion were given in 1977 by S.J. Konturek and 11 years later by M.V. Singer (1988) signaling progress in this field.

Parallel to the constant interest in the regulation was the study of the biochemistry and secretion of the pancreatic enzymes and their synthesis. At most meetings there were sessions with papers on these topics. In 1983, a large symposium was held in Verona with the title 'Pancreatic Proteases and Antiproteases in Physiological and Patho-

Table 3. Symposia, round tables, working sessions, panel discussions and their chairmen at the meetings of the EPC

1968	Prague	Panel Discussion: Surgical treatment of pancreatitis	W. Hess
1969	Göttingen	Panel Discussion: Standardization of pancreatic function tests	W. Creutzfeldt
1975	Toulouse	Pathophysiology and treatment of experimental and human acute pancreatitis	T.T. White
		Gastrointestinal hormones and related peptides	S.J. Konturek
		Regulation and adaptation of pancreatic secretion	K.G. Wormsley
		Endoscopic retrograde catheterism of the papilla	P.B. Cotton
1977	Dublin	Panel: Current problems in pancreatic inflammatory disease	
		Excitation-contraction coupling in the pancreas	J. Scott
		Experimental pancreatitis	D.J. Hingerty
		Experimental studies using alcohol and its metabolites on the pancreas	J.M. Fitzpatrick
1982	Essen	Controversies in medicine: The treatment of acute pancreatitis	R. Ammann
1983	Verona	Pancreatic proteases and antiproteases in phys. and path. conditions	A. Ribet
		Controversies in medicine: Pancreatic cancer, diagnostics and therapeutics	K.G. Wormsley
1984	Cascais	Pancreatic secretion	J. Christophe
		Pathogenesis of chronic alcoholic pancreatitis	J.C. Bode
1987	Marseilles	Acute pancreatitis – pseudocysts	H.G. Beger
1988	Budapest	Pain in chronic pancreatitis – causes and management	H. Goebell
1989	Glasgow	The role of interventional radiology and other imaging modalities in pancreatic disease	C.W. Imrie
		Pancreatic disease of the Atlantic salmon	A.K. Foulis
1991	Lund	Report on diagnosis of exocrine pancreatic disease	I. Ihse
1992	Ulm	The role of somatostatin and octreotide in pancreatic disease	R. Arnold
		The role of enzyme treatment in pancreatic disease	H.G. Beger
1993	Paris	Chloride channels in normal and pathological pancreas	O.H. Petersen
		Cystic tumors of the pancreas	A.L. Warshaw
1994	Bologna	New therapeutic approaches in chronic pancreatitis	H. Worning
1995	Barcelona	Pancreatic cancer	C.D. Johnson
		Acinar islet cell interaction	J.B. Jansen
		Laparoscopy as a new tool of diagnosis and treatment of pancreatic disease	H.G. Beger
1996	Mannheim	New treatment of pancreatic cancer	E. DiMagno
		Islet transplantation – dream or reality?	U.R. Fölsch
		Cytokines in pancreatic diseases	H. Goebell
1997	London	Reactive oxygen radicals	L. Fernandez-Cruz
1998	Thessaloniki	Imaging methods in pancreatic disease	J.B. Jansen
1999	Lüneburg	Molecular biology in pancreatic cancer	N. Lemoine
		Satellite Meeting: Pancreatic enzyme therapy following surgical procedures in the gastrointestinal tract; half day	P.G. Lankisch
		Basic Science Satellite Symposium: Frontiers in pancreatic physiology; 1 day (Advisory Board: G. Adler, A. Fink, L. Miller, S. Muallem, J.Williams)	M. Case and P.G. Lankisch
2000	Kiel	Prophylactic antibiotics and early nutrition in acute pancreatitis	C. Beglinger
		Cytokines and acute pancreatitis	A. Andren-Sandberg
2001	Toulouse	Future prospects for the medical management of adenocarcinoma of the exocrine pancreas	P. Ruszniewski
		Role of pancreatic surgery	H.G. Beger
2002	Heidelberg	Pancreas development and tumor cell biology	B. Greenhalf
		Clinical controversies in acute pancreatitis	M.W. Büchler
		Clinical controversies in chronic pancreatitis	H.G. Beger
		What's new in imaging and endoscopic treatment?	J.E. Cunha
		Pancreas cell physiology and pancreatitis cell biology	G. Adler
		Pancreatic surgery – how it's done	I. Ihse
		Clinical controversies in pancreatic cancer	M. Brennan
		Acute pancreatitis – indications for surgery	J.P. Neoptolemos
2003	Liverpool	Clinical advances in pancreatic cancer	N. Lemoine
		Clinical controversies in acute pancreatitis	R. Charnley
		Pathophysiology of acute pancreatitis	M. Bhatia
		Basic science	O.H. Petersen
		Clinical chronic pancreatitis	R. Malfertheiner
		International Pancreas Basic Science Workshop; 1 day	O.H. Petersen
2004	Padova	Diabetes in pancreatic diseases	J. Permert
		Endocrine pancreatic tumors	K. Öberg
		Pancreatic cancer	C. Johnson
		Signal transduction in pancreatic islet cells	T. Pozzan

On average, 4–8 researchers were involved. We apologize for any omissions that might have occurred. Symposium is used as a synonym for panel, round table and symposium.

Table 4. Invited lectures (L) and symposia (S) dealing with hormones, nerves and regulation of pancreatic secretion

Structure and function of hormones (secretin, pancreozymin, gastrin, cerulein)	L	J.E. Jorpes, V. Mutt, J.S. Morley, A. Anastasi, A.A. Harper	1968
New aspects of hydrelatic secretion of the exocrine pancreas	L	T. Scratcherd	1975
New aspects of enzyme secretion	L	J. Meldolesi	1975
Regulation and adaptation of pancreatic secretion	S	Toulouse	1975
Gastrointestinal hormones and related peptides	S	Toulouse	1977
Secretin: Physiological and clinical implications	L	K.G. Wormsley	1979
Intestinal hormones and exocrine pancreas	L	O. Schaffalitzky de Muckadell	1981
Pancreatic proteases and antiproteases in physiological and pathological conditions	S	Verona	1983
Pancreatic secretion	S	Cascais	1984
Ion channels and pumps in pancreatic acinar cells	L	O.H. Petersen	1987
Pharmacology of the pancreas	L	H. Goebell	1988
Pancreatic basic research and clinical sciences	L	L. Gullo	1988
New aspects in the neural regulation of pancreatic function	L	M.V. Singer	1988
Evidence of hormonal status of somatostatin 28	L	J.W. Ensick	1990
Gene regulation of pancreatic enzymes in pancreatitis	L	J.C. Dagorn	1990
The role of somatostatin and octreotide in pancreatic disease	S	Ulm	1992
Pancreatic colipase: Structural and physiological aspects	L	G. Erlanson-Albertsson	1994
Neurohormonal control of pancreatic secretion	L	T. Solomon	1996
Neural changes in pancreatic disease	L	D. Bockman	1996
Nitric oxide and pancreatic secretion	L	J.J. Calvo	1998
Regulation of pancreatic secretion	L	P. Layer	1998
Protein kinase signaling cascades induced by pancreatic secretagogues	L	U.R. Fölsch	1998
Control of pancreatic duct cell secretion	L	B. Argent	2002

logical Condition'; 'The Amino Acid Transport in the Pancreas' was a lecture by G. Mann in 1994, on colipase by G. Erlansson-Albertsson in 1994 and J.C. Dagorn reported first on the gene regulation of pancreatic enzymes in 1990. The secretion of water and electrolytes from the ducts was also of special interest in some lectures (T. Scratcherd, 1975 and B. Argent, 2002).

The role of the newly discovered hormone somatostatin in the pancreas was discussed in a working session under the moderation of S. Bloom with 4 speakers in Toulouse in 1975 and later at a symposium in Ulm in 1992, covering also aspects of possible use in the treatment of pancreatic inflammation via the inhibitory effect on pancreatic secretion.

Cell Biology of the Pancreas (table 5)

The development of new methods for the study of intracellular events in the 1970s and 1980s opened the field of cell biology also to the pancreas (receptors, calcium signaling, patch-clamp technique, cell culture). The interest of basic scientists was raised by the fact that the pancreatic acinar cell and the duct cell system offer models for the study of fundamental biological processes. This was reflected also in the meetings of the EPC over many years (see table 5) until today.

The events of stimulus-secretion coupling (M. Case, 1988), the study of ion channels and pumps (O.H. Petersen, 1987; symposium in Paris, 1993; workshop in Liverpool, 2003), the role of calcium in these processes (O.H. Petersen, 1992; M. Case, 1992; workshop, 2003) were the main topics.

In the 1970s, the analysis of receptors on the acinar and duct cells started. Major contributions to lectures and symposia came from J. Christophe (1978), H.J. Geuze (1986), W. Creutzfeldt (1992), J.A. Williams (1993), J. Jensen (1994) and others. In 1992, Creutzfeldt analyzed our knowledge on CCK-receptor antagonists.

At the 31st meeting in Lüneburg a whole day was dedicated to basic science ('Frontiers in Pancreatic Physiology') organized by Maynard Case and Paul Lankisch with the help of G. Adler, A. Fink, L. Miller, S. Muallem and J. Williams. The topics were regulation, signaling, acinar secretory pathway, duct cell secretion and gene expression.

The ongoing interest in the field of cell biology was documented only recently at the meeting in Liverpool in 2003. A symposium on 'Basic Science' gave information on the progress in this field with J.A. Williams (new insights in the working of the acinar cell), Y. Maryama (G-binding proteins), B. Argent (secretion by pancreatic duct cells)

Table 5. Invited lectures (L) and symposia (S) dealing with special topics in basic science

Intracellular events			
Excitation-contraction coupling	S	Dublin	1977
Stimulus-secretion coupling, calcium signaling			
Ion channels and pumps in pancreatic acinar cells	L	O.H. Petersen	1987
Development of secretory polarity in the pancreatic acinar cell	L	J.D. Jamieson	1987
Critical evaluation of results obtained in the field of stimulus-secretion coupling	L	M. Case	1988
Molecular aspects of calcium signaling	L	O.H. Petersen	1992
Secretory polarity	L	M. Case	1992
Chloride channels and transporters in normal and pathological cells (Petersen, Argent, Schulz, deJonge)	S	Paris, 4 speakers	1993
The role of calcium in pancreatic secretion	L	O.H. Petersen	1998
Intracellular signaling in pancreatic acinar cells	L	S. Muallem	1999
Tyrosine phosphorylation and dephosphorylation in pancreatic signal transduction	L	L. Buscail	1999
Regulation of pancreatic protein synthesis	L	J.A Williams	1999
Nitric oxide and pancreatic function	S	London	1997
Basic science: Acinar cell, G-binding proteins, duct cells, calcium (Williams, Maruyama, Argent, Tepikin)	S	Liverpool, 4 speakers	2003
Intern. Basic Science Workshop: Secretion, calcium, etc.	S	Liverpool, 13 speakers	2003
Receptors			
Hormone responsiveness of the plasma membrane of pancreatic cells	L	J. Christophe	1978
Molecular and structural aspects of pancreatic adaptation	L	H. Kern	1982
Sorting of membrane receptors in the secretory and endocytotic pathway	L	H.J. Geuze	1986
From receptors of VIP-and CCK families to G protein in acinar cell line	L	J. Christophe	1992
CCK receptor antagonists	L	W. Creutzfeldt	1992
Cytokine-growth factor receptor interaction	L	W. Schmiegel	1992
New developments in the control mechanisms of pancreatic acinar cells	L	J.A. Williams	1993
Molecular biology of pancreatic receptors	L	J. Jensen	1994
Gene regulation of pancreatic cell receptors	L	H.C. Weber	1996
CCK_A receptors coupled to multiple signal transduction systems in pancreatic acini	L	Y. Tsunoda	1999
Molecular basis of cholecystokinin receptor binding	L	J. Miller	1999
Applied cell biology			
Cell biology of acute pancreatitis	L	M.L. Steer	1992
Pancreas cell biology and pancreatitis (Adrian, Iovanna, Graf, Saluja, Petersen, Göke)	S	Heidelberg, 6 speakers	2002

and A. Tepikin (calcium signaling in the acinar cell). At the same meeting over a whole day the 'International Pancreas Basic Science Workshop – Beyond Frontiers' with 17 speakers showed the unbroken interest in these fields.

Methods of cell biology were also applied to the pathogenesis of acute pancreatitis (M. Steer, 1992) and this was, furthermore, the topic of a symposium in 2002 (regulation of protein synthesis, pancreatic cell response to stress, pancreatic stress proteins, intracellular colocalization, calcium signaling and acute pancreatitis). Cytokine studies started in the 1990s, especially the relation to growth factor receptor (W. Schmiegel, 1992), in pancreatic cancer and in acute pancreatitis (panel on cytokines and acute pancreatitis, 2000, see table 8).

Endocrine-Exocrine Relationship (table 6)

The role of the endocrine pancreas was highlighted in 1979 for the first time at an EPC meeting in a lecture by S. Bloom. The endocrine pancreas attracted attention itself, in relation to the exocrine pancreas and clinically with endocrine tumors (E. Solcia, 1983; D. Winick, 1990; S.W. Lamberts, 1993; P. Serup, 2001). The interaction between the islet cells and exocrine tissue (W.J. Malaisse, 1982; V.L. Go, 1984; a panel on 'Acinar-Islet Cell Interaction', Barcelona, 1995) but also the enteroinsular axis (W. Creutzfeldt, 1981) were issues of lectures.

Total pancreatectomy and its pathophysiological consequences attained attraction (W. Creutzfeldt, 1981) as well as pancreas transplantation (D. Sutherland, 1994).

Table 6. Invited lectures (L) and symposia (S) dealing with the endocrine pancreas and relations to the exocrine pancreas

The endocrine pancreas	L	S. Bloom	1979
Entero-insular axis, physiological and clinical aspects	L	W. Creutzfeldt	1981
Total pancreatectomy, indications and pathophysiological consequences	L	W. Creutzfeldt	1981
Cellular heterogeneity and interrelationship in pancreatic islet and acinar tissue	L	W.J. Malaisse	1982
The endocrine tumors of the pancreas	L	E. Solcia	1983
Pancreas endo-exocrine interaction	L	V.L. Go	1984
Endocrine tumors of the pancreas, clinics, diagnosis and treatment	L	D. Wynick	1990
Evidence of the hormonal status of S-28 on endo- and exocrine pancreatic functions in man	L	J.W. Ensinck	1990
Nutritional (tropical) diabetes and pancreatitis	L	K.G. Alberti	1990
Recent advances in the imaging of pancreatic endocrine tumors	L	S.W. Lamberts	1993
Pancreas transplantation – present and future	L	D. Sutherland	1994
Acinar-islet cell interaction (Jensen, v. Schoenfeld, Figarella)	S	Barcelona, 3 speakers	1995
Islet transplantation – dream or reality	S	Mannheim, 7 speakers	1996
Pancreatic beta cell proliferation	L	A. Sjöholm	2000
Control of pancreatic endocrine lineage determination	L	P. Serup	2001
Epidemiology of pancreatic exocrine insufficiency and diabetes mellitus	L	W. Rathmann	2002
Signal transduction in pancreatic islet cells	S	Padova, 4 speakers	2004
Endocrine pancreatic tumors	S	Padova, 5 speakers	2004
Diabetes in pancreatic diseases	S	Padova, 6 speakers	2004

Table 7. Invited lectures (L) dealing with nutrition and the pancreas

The gastrointestinal handling of different meals in man	L	H.O. Lagerlöf	1974
Geographical pancreatitis	L	H. Sarles	1977
Molecular and structural aspects of exocrine pancreatic adaptation to changing functional demands	L	H. Kern	1982
Pathophysiology and treatment of pancreatic maldigestion and meal absorption	L	E. DiMagno	1983
Nutritional factors and pancreatic cancer	L	H. Worning	1988
Nutritional (tropical) diabetes and pancreatitis	L	K.G. Alberti	1990
Nutrition in pancreatitis – the role in pathophysiology and treatment	L	J.S. Scolapio	1999
Pancreatic enzymes and digestion	L	C. Erlanson-Albertsson	1998

Nutrition and the Pancreas (table 7)

Nutritional factors are important in the etiology of chronic pancreatitis. H. Sarles reported in a lecture on geographical pancreatitis in Africa and India, mainly Kerala, as did K.G. Alberti in 1990. A combination of certain foodstuffs (cassava) and protein malnutrition at that time seemed to be decisive factors for a clinical picture like chronic pancreatitis with calcification but without alcohol intake.

In the meantime, the detection that 50% of the patients with tropical pancreatitis carry SPINK 1 mutations also classifies this disease entity as an inherited disease.

The pancreas also has the potential to adapt to different food. This finding of possible adaptation in the 1980s stimulated many experimental studies (H. Kern, 1982 on molecular and structural aspects of exocrine pancreatic adaptation). H. Worning summarized the knowledge about nutritional factors in pancreatic cancer (1988). Maldigestion due to pancreatic insufficiency was an important issue in lectures by H.O. Lagerlöf (1974), E. DiMagno (1983) and J.S. Scolapio (1999).

Acute Pancreatitis (table 8)

At all EPC meetings the issue of the etiology, pathogenesis, pathology, diagnosis and treatment of acute pancreatitis were important topics in experimental work and clinical presentations (symposia in Prague, 1968; Toulouse, 1975; Dublin, 1977). In 1982, a panel discussion took place in Essen on the treatment of acute pancreatitis and controversial views (conservative against surgical). A similar discussion was held at a symposium in 2002 in Heidelberg, showing that the problem was still unsolved. In 1988, C. Imrie gave a lecture on terminology, pathogenesis and therapy of acute pancreatitis and laid ground for future work and systematic analysis.

Table 8. Invited lectures (L) and symposia (S) dealing with experimental and clinical acute pancreatitis

Panel: Surgical treatment of pancreatitis	S	Prague	1968
Pathophysiology and treatment of experimental and human pancreatitis	S	Toulouse	1975
Current problems in pancreatic inflammatory disease	S	Dublin	1977
Controversies in medicine: The treatment of acute pancreatitis	S	Essen, 4 speakers	1982
Pancreatitis: Terminology, pathogenesis, therapy	L	C. Imrie	1988
Acute pancreatitis and pseudocysts (Beger, Büchler, Engelholm, Henriksen, Imrie, Malfertheimer, Sahel, Sarles)	S	Marseilles, 8 participants	1987
Cell regeneration in acute pancreatitis	L	G. Adler	1990
Interventional therapeutic approaches for complications of pancreatic abscess	L	S. Gerzof	1990
Cell biology of acute pancreatitis	L	M.L. Steer	1992
Biliary pancreatitis – Facts and fashion	L	J.P. Neoptolemos	1992
Free radicals and tissue damage	L	B. Haliwell	1993
The acute pancreatitis patient with extended necrosis	L	C. Frey	1994
Cytokines in pancreatic disease	S	Mannheim	1996
Nitric oxide and pancreatic function	S	London	1997
Bradykinin and pancreatic dysfunction	S	London	1997
Intracellular events in acute pancreatitis	L	G. Mann	1998
Management of acute pancreatitis	L	P.G. Lankisch	1998
Activation peptides of pancreatic proteases	L	A. Borgström	1999
Premature pancreatic protease activation – mechanisms	L	M. Lerch	1999
Cytokines and chemokines – multiple players and a single goal	L	A. Saluja	1999
The role of the gut in acute pancreatitis	L	M. McMahon	1999
Laparoscopic interventions for pancreatitis	L	C. McKay	1999
Early nutrition in acute pancreatitis and prophylactic antibiotics	S	Kiel, 5 participants	2000
Cytokines and pancreatitis	S	Kiel, 3 participants	2000
TGF beta – impact on acute and chronic pancreatitis	L	J. van Laethem	2000
Gene expression of cytokines in acute pancreatitis	L	J.C. Dagorn	2000
Acute pancreatitis and cytokines	L	J.L. van Laethen	2001
Evaluation of trypsinogen activation peptide as a prognostic marker in the assessment of acute pancreatitis	L	J.P. Neoptolemos	2001
Molecular pathology of trypsinogen in acute pancreatitis	L	J.M. Chen	2001
Attack or defense in acute pancreatitis	L	M. Lerch	2002
Do we need prognostic scores or markers?	L	J. Schmidt	2002
Acute pancreatitis: Indications for surgery – IAP guidelines development	S	Heidelberg, 11 participants	2002 (together with the IAP)
Microcirculatory dysfunction in acute pancreatitis	L	B. Vollmar	2002
Clinical controversies in acute pancreatitis (contrast-enhanced CT, prophylactic antibiotics, enteral feeding yes or no)	S	Heidelberg, 9 participants	2002
Pancreas cell physiology and pancreatitis	S	Heidelberg, 9 participants	2002
Clinical controversies in acute pancreatitis (early mortality, prophylactic antibiotics, minimally invasive necrosectomy, interventional radiology)	S	Liverpool, 11 participants	2003
Bile acids cause death of pancreatic acinar cells	L	S. Muallem	2003

In the 1990s, studies on the cell biology of acute pancreatitis gave new ideas for experimental research. The role of lysosomes was investigated by M. Steer (1992), free radicals and tissue damage by B. Haliwell (1993) and the role of cytokines in the disease process was looked at in a symposium in 2000 and in a lecture by J.L. van Laethen in 2001. It is important to say that the discovery of trypsinogen mutations by D. Whitcomb as a genetic basis in hereditary pancreatitis also led to a better understanding of the pathogenesis of acute pancreatitis. D. Whitcomb gave state-of-the-art lectures on this topic in 1998 and 2003 (see table 14). Molecular pathology of trypsinogen in pancreatitis was also reported by J.M. Chen in 2001, and microcirculatory dysfunction in acute pancreatitis was discussed in a lecture by B. Vollmar in 2002. Important issues of pancreatic cell physiology in acute pancreatitis were summarized only recently at a symposium in Heidelberg in 2002.

Items of clinical care in acute pancreatitis turned up from time to time in lectures, i.e. on 'Biliary Pancreati-

Table 9. Invited lectures (L) and symposia (S) dealing with experimental and clinical chronic pancreatitis

Physiopathology of alcoholic chronic pancreatitis	L	H. Sarles	1975
Pathogenesis of chronic alcoholic pancreatitis	S	Cascais, 8 participants	1984
Pancreatic structure – a broad view	L	D.E. Bockman	1984
Pancreatic lithiasis	L	H. Sarles	1988
Pain in chronic pancreatitis – cause and management	S	Budapest, 12 participants	1988
Gene regulation of pancreatic enzymes in pancreatitis	L	J.C. Dagorn	1990
Staging of chronic pancreatitis to optimize therapy and prognosis	L	R. Ammann	1991
The role of enzyme treatment in pancreatic disease	S	Ulm, 8 participants	1992
Inhibition of calcium salt crystallization and lithiasis in the digestive tract and the kidney	L	H. Sarles	1993
Does acute alcoholic pancreatitis occur in the absence of chronic pancreatic lesions?	L	M.V. Singer	1994
New therapeutic approaches in chronic pancreatitis	S	Bologna	1994
Pancreatic enzyme therapy following surgical procedures in the gastrointestinal tract	S	Lüneburg, 11 participants	1999
Pancreatic exocrine insufficiency and diabetes mellitus	L	W. Rathmann	1999
DBTC – pancreatitis: A new experimental model for chronic pancreatitis?	L	J. Merkord	1999
Alcohol-induced acute pancreatitis – does it exist?	L	M.V. Singer	1999
Autoimmune chronic pancreatitis – a relevant entity?	L	M. Tiemann	1999
Pancreatic enzyme substitution – does particle size make a difference?	L	J. Mössner	1999
Pancreatic stellate cells – new players in pancreatic fibrosis?	L	G. Adler	1999
TGF beta – an autocrine loop for stellate cells?	L	M.L. Kruse	1999
100 years of pancreatic enzyme substitution – present state and future developments	L	J. Moreau	2000
Pancreatic stellate cells in human and experimental pancreatic fibrosis	L	J.S. Wilson	2000
Porcine, bovine, fungal or bacterial lipase – benefits and deficits	L	P. Layer	2001
SPINK 1 mutations in chronic pancreatitis	L	H. Witt	2001
Molecular pathology of trypsinogen in pancreatitis	L	J.M. Chen	2001
Problem of pain in chronic pancreatitis	L	E. DiMagno	2001
Clinical controversies in chronic pancreatitis	S	Heidelberg, 11 participants	2002
What can genetics tell us about the pathophysiology of chronic pancreatitis	L	H. Witt	2003
Clinical chronic pancreatitis	S	Liverpool, 8 participants	2003
The problem of advanced chronic pancreatitis	L	M.W. Büchler	2003
Molecular pathology of chronic pancreatitis	L	H. Friess	2004
On the role of stellate cells in fibrogenesis	L	M.G. Bachem	2004
Role of surgery in chronic pancreatitis	L	M.W. Büchler	2004

tis – Facts and Fashions' (J. Neoptolemos, 1992) and on 'Early Nutrition and Prophylactic Antibiotics' (a panel in Heidelberg, 2002). Clinicians have always been very interested in prognostic scores and markers in acute pancreatitis. They have been absolutely essential in prospective trials since the work of Ranson in the 1970s and have been the topic of a summarizing lecture in 2002 (J. Schmidt).

Chronic Pancreatitis (table 9)

Several approaches have been made to develop an internationally accepted classification of pancreatitis, first of the chronic variety, but also of the different stages of acute inflammation. On the initiative of Henri Sarles a first classification was defined in Marseilles in 1963. Another approach was undertaken in 1984 in Marseilles again to develop the principles further. These classifications were based on pathology, on pancreatic function and on etiology. Chronic calcifying pancreatitis played an important role in relation to alcohol intake.

Another classification of chronic pancreatitis was formulated on the initiative of M. Sarner and P.B. Cotton in Cambridge in 1983. It was based on the alterations of the pancreatic ducts which are visualized by ERP. These classifications, incomplete as they were, have contributed greatly to the understanding of pancreatitis. In 1991, R. Ammann gave a lecture on 'Staging of Chronic Pancreatitis to Optimize Therapy and Prognosis'.

The main poison for the pancreas seems to be alcohol. In 1975, Henri Sarles presented 'The Physiopathology of Alcoholic Pancreatitis' in a lecture. He developed the hypothesis that a defect in the secretion of a calcium-binding protein (pancreatic stone protein, PSP) is responsible for the precipitation of calcium salts in the ducts, which in turn lead to chronic pancreatitis. The discussions on the existence and possible role of PSP have been ongoing

Table 10. Invited lectures (L) and symposia (S) dealing with function tests and imaging of the pancreas

Function tests	Standardization of pancreatic function tests	S	Göttingen	1969
	The gastrointestinal handling of different meals in man	L	H.O. Lagerlöf	1974
	Are function tests still useful as diagnostic tools in diseases of the exocrine pancreas?	L	R. Ammann	1988
	Why and how to search for pancreatic insufficiency	L	B. Glasbrenner	2001
Endoscopy and imaging	New aspects of endoscopy in pancreatology	L	G.S. Nagy, L. Safrany	1988
	Endosopic sonography for the pancreas – does it help in the diagnosis and management of pancreatic disease?	L	T. Rösch	1990
	Interventional therapeutic approaches for complications of pancreatic abscess	L	S. Gerzof	1990
	The role of interventional radiology and other imaging modalities in pancreatic disease	S	Glasgow	1989
	Imaging methods in pancreatic disease	S	Thessaloniki	1998
	Magnetic resonance pancreatography (MRP)	L	J.F. Riemann	2000
	Positron emission tomography (PET)	L	W. Weber	2000
	Endosonography	L	L. Buscail	2000
	Laparoscopy as a new tool for diagnosis and treatment of pancreatic disease	S	Heidelberg	2002
	What's new in imaging and endoscopic treatment	S	Heidelberg	2002
	Laparoscopic surgery in pancreatic diseases	L	L. Fernandez-Cruz	2004

at the EPC meetings for many years. In 1984, a symposium in Cascais on the pathogenesis of chronic alcoholic pancreatitis tried to further elucidate the problem. Direct toxic damage to the pancreatic tissue by alcohol without involvement of altered secretion of PSP was a point of discussion. The question of whether acute alcoholic pancreatitis can occur in the absence of chronic pancreatic lesions was discussed by M.V. Singer in a lecture (1994). The question could not be finally answered. The problem of PSP was finally settled, by stating that it is not the ultimate explanation for the development of chronic calcifying pancreatitis. Obviously PSP does not exist in the proposed molecular form.

More practical problems of chronic pancreatitis, like pain management (symposium in Budapest, 1988; lecture by E. DiMagno, 2001) and the enzyme treatment of maldigestion (symposium in Ulm, 1992; also in Bologna, 1994, and in Lüneburg, 1999, and state-of-the-art lectures by J. Moreau, 2000 and by P. Layer, 2001) demonstrated the widespread interest in these questions at the EPC meetings over the years. In Heidelberg in 2002 and in Liverpool in 2003, symposia took place on clinical controversies in chronic pancreatitis (conservative and surgical treatment).

Function Tests and Imaging of the Pancreas (table 10)

Over the 40 years, from 1965 until now, some progress has been made concerning the diagnostic tools as regards diseases of the pancreas. The evaluation of enzyme levels in the serum (amylase, lipase) and the measurement of pancreatic exocrine function remained the basic principles.

Great efforts were made to develop standardized tests for the function of the exocrine pancreas. Special tubes (Lagerlöf tube, double lumen, double balloon tube) and the application of test meals (Lundh test) or of intravenous standardized doses of secretin and pancreozymin/cerulein allowed the controlled suction of duodenal juice. The analysis of bicarbonate and enzymes in the basic and stimulated duodenal (pancreatic) juice made it possible to define normal secretion and different grades of impairment as pancreatic exocrine insufficiency in chronic pancreatitis (symposium on 'Standardization of Pancreatic Function Tests', Göttingen, 1969). Also the concentration of chymotrypsin in stool (and later of elastase) was used as a parameter for the function of the exocrine pancreas. In 1988, R. Ammann asked in a lecture: 'Are Function Tests Useful as Diagnostic Tools in Diseases of the Exocrine Pancreas?' L.B. Glasbrenner discussed the same question in 2001 in a lecture. The answer is: yes, they are.

Scintigraphy of the pancreas using ^{75}Se-methionine started being used in the 1970s but was soon obsolete, because ultrasonography, computerized tomography and endoscopic retrograde cholangiopancreaticography with contrast medium (ERCP) offered better methods of imaging. ERCP became a leading tool, also for interventional treatment (stenting, stone extraction). All these methods were frequent topics at the EPC meetings in Free Paper Sessions, but also in lectures (L. Safrany, 1988; S. Gerzof, 1990; symposium, 2002). The development of endoscopic ultrasound imaging (T. Rösch, 1990; L. Buscail, 2000), of magnetic resonance imaging/magnetic resonance chol-

Table 11. Invited lectures (L) and symposia (S) dealing with pancreatic development and cell growth

Interrelation of secretory and trophic responses in the exocrine pancreas	L	N. Vaysse	1988
Cytokine growth factor receptor interaction	L	W. Schmiegel	1992
Growth factor receptors and growth of pancreatic cancer	L	M. Korc	1992
Pancreatic cell growth – facts and fashion	L	N. Vaysse	1992
New developments in the control mechanisms of pancreatic acinar cells	L	J.A. Williams	1993
TGF beta and regulated transcription factors in pancreatic development and cancer	L	R. Urrutia	2001
Pancreatic development and tumor cell biology (Bockman, Mayerle, Tosh, Wagner, Fries)	S	Heidelberg, 5 speakers	2002
Apoptosis in pancreatic pathology	L	J.J. Dagorn	1998
Pancreatic development	L	L.M. Wagner	2000
Complex in vitro systems	L	H. Kalthoff	2000

angiopancreatography (MRCP; J. Riemann, 2000) and also of positron emission tomography (PET; W. Weber, 2000) were critically discussed as a new way to diagnosis at the EPC meetings.

Pancreatic Development and Cell Growth (table 11)
The trophic behavior of the pancreas gained great interest with respect to the development of cancer. In 1988, a lecture by Nicole Vaysse dealt with the 'Interrelationship of Secretory and Trophic Responses in the Exocrine Pancreas'. In 1992, she was invited to give another lecture on this topic ('Pancreatic Cell Growth – Facts and Fashions'). W. Schmiegel (1992) investigated cytokine-growth factor receptor interactions and M. Korc (1992) growth factor receptors and the growth of pancreatic cancer. Also transcription factors in pancreatic development and cancer were investigated (lecture by R. Urrutia, 2001). In 2002, at Heidelberg a symposium on 'Pancreas Development and Tumor Cell Biology' with 5 speakers tried to summarize the knowledge.

Pancreatic Cancer: Experimental Work (table 12)
Although much experimental work on pancreatic cancer was presented over the last 40 years at the EPC meetings, there were only real new results with new methods of molecular biology and genetic research. Two state-of-the-art lectures were held in the early 1990s (F. Mitelman, 1991; G. Klöppel, 1992) and then again in 2000. Transgenic models for pancreatic cancer were developed (R. Schmid, 2000 and 2002), TGF-β and cancer were investigated (R. Urrutia, 2001), and the molecular genetics of pancreatic cancer (N. Lemoine, 2000) and the functional and structural characteristics of cultured pancreatic cancer cells (G. Klöppel, 2000) were addressed in lectures. A whole symposium was dedicated to pancreas development and tumor cell biology in Heidelberg in 2002. Gene therapy of pancreatic cancer was discussed by M. Löhr and by L. Buscail in 2001 in lectures.

Pancreatic Cancer: Clinical Work (table 13)
In the EPC meetings there were regular Free Paper Sessions on the clinical problems of cancer, diagnostic and therapeutic aspects. Lectures and panel rounds were invited to summarize our knowledge. The first extended report was given in 1981 by K.G. Wormsley ('Experimental and Clinical Problems of Pancreatic Carcinogenesis'), diagnostic and therapeutic problems were the topic of a symposium in Verona in 1983 and again in Barcelona in 1995. Members of another panel gave a talk in Heidelberg in 2002 and in Liverpool in 2003. This intensification of discussion rounds on cancer in comparison to former years shows that in recent years there has been considerable hope for better diagnosis and treatment.

In lectures the topics of nutritional aspects (H. Worning, 1988), of epidemiology (C. LaVecchia, 1994), of radiotherapy (R. Dobelbower, 1990), of early clinical signs for diagnosis (L. Gullo, 2002) and of chemotherapeutic agents for the treatment (E. van Cutsem, 2000) have been presented by invited speakers. A special symposium was organized on the question of familial pancreatic cancer in Toulouse 2001 (3 speakers). In this context it is interesting that in the frame of the EPC since 1995 a European study group for pancreatic cancer has been founded, which runs several trials (ESPAC) and has had sessions at all EPC meetings since then.

Genetic Studies and the Pancreas (table 14)
Hereditary pancreatitis has been known for a long time in families with acute and chronic disease. Also, the sporadic occurrence of chronic calcifying pancreatitis in very young people without alcohol intake points in this direction (Ammann). Hereditary pancreatitis was the topic of

Table 12. Invited lectures (L) and symposia (S) dealing with experimental pancreatic cancer

Potential value of chromosome investigation in pancreatic cancer	L	F. Mitelman	1991
Pancreatic cancer: What makes it so different from other GI carcinomas	L	G. Klöppel	1992
Molecular biology of pancreatic tumors (genetics, nucleic acid fingerprinting, etc.)	S	Mannheim	1996
Pathology and treatment of pancreatic cancer	S	London	1997
Antimitogenic signaling via somatostatin A receptors	L	N. Vaysse	1998
Resistance to apoptosis	L	H. Kalthoff	1999
Functional and structural characteristics of cultured pancreatic cancer cells	L	G. Klöppel	2000
Transgenic models for pancreatic cancer	L	R. Schmid	2000
Xenotransplantation model of pancreatic cancer	L	F.X. Real	2000
Molecular genetics of pancreatic cancer	L	N. Lemoine	2000
Complex in vitro systems	L	H. Kalthoff	2000
Gene therapy for pancreatic cancer – intratumoral targeted chemotherapy	L	M. Löhr	2001
Gene therapy for pancreatic cancer – gene correction by Ssst?	L	L. Buscail	2001
TGF beta and regulated transcription factors in pancreatic development and cancer	L	R. Urrutia	2001
Pathogenesis of early pancreatic cancer	L	R. Schmid	2002
Pancreas development and tumor cell biology (development, cell contact regulation, transdifferentiation, murine tumor model, adaptation)	S	Heidelberg, 5 speakers	2002
Apoptosis signaling in pancreatic cancer cells: Suitable targets for therapy	L	H. Kalthoff	2004
Targeting K-ras mutations and telomerase in pancreatic cancer by therapeutic vaccines	L	G. Gaudernack	2004

Table 13. Invited lectures (L) and symposia (S) dealing with clinical pancreatic cancer

Experimental and clinical problems of pancreatic carcinogenesis	L	K.G. Wormsley	1981
Pancreatic cancer: Diagnostic and therapeutic problems	S	Verona, 6 participants	1983
Treatment of pancreatic cancer	L	H. Joyeux	1984
Nutritional factors and pancreatic cancer	L	H. Worning	1988
Radiotherapy of pancreatic cancer	L	R.R. Dobelbower	1990
Progress in diagnosis and treatment pancreatic carcinoma	L	M. Trede	1992
Epidemiology of pancreatic cancer	L	C. La Vecchia	1994
Pancreatic cancer (endoscopic ultrasonography, laparoscopy, resection, second look)	S	Barcelona, 4 speakers	1995
New treatment of pancreatic cancer (somatostatin, gemcitabine, vaccines, chemotherapy, surgery)	S	Mannheim	1996
Intraductal papillary mucinous tumors	L	M. Cremer	1998
Prodrug activation – a new treatment for pancreatic cancer?	L	M. Löhr	1999
Immunological changes in pancreatic carcinoma – basis for novel strategies	L	F. Gansauge	1999
Metastasis formation in pancreatic cancer	L	H. Friess	1999
Novel chemotherapeutic agents for the treatment of pancreatic cancer	L	E. van Cutsem	2000
Familial pancreatic cancer, EUROPAC	S	Toulouse, 3 speakers	2001
Future prospects for the medical management of adenocarcinoma of the exocrine pancreas (CT, MRI, endoscopic ultrasonography, surgery, radiotherapy, chemotherapy)	S	Toulouse, 4 speakers	2001
Are there early clinical signs for pancreatic carcinoma?	L	L. Gullo	2001
Clinical controversies in pancreatic cancer (stents vs. surgery, resection head of p. pylorus preserving vs. standard Whipple resection, Pap, Reber, Kawarada, Gouma, Permert, Warshaw)	S	Heidelberg, 6 speakers	2002
Pathogenesis of early pancreatic cancer	L	R. Schmid	2002
The role of case load and experience in pancreas cancer surgery	L	H. Obertop	2002
Dominant signaling pathways in pancreatic cancer progression	L	R. Urrutia	2003
Clinical advances in pancreatic cancer (gene therapy, improved survival, adjuvant therapy)	S	Liverpool, 3 speakers	2003
Physiopathology of cachexia in pancreatic cancer	L	S. Wyke	2004
Pancreatic cancer (gene therapy, chemotherapy, radiotherapy, Vaysse, Löhr, Uomo, Heinemann, Alessio)	S	Padova, 5 speakers	2004

Table 14. Invited lectures (L) and symposia (S) dealing with genetics and the pancreas and with cystic fibrosis

Gene regulation of pancreatic enzymes in pancreatitis	L	J.C. Dagorn	1990
Potential value of chromosome investigation in pancreatic cancer	L	F. Mitelman	1991
Hereditary pancreatitis	L	D. Whitcomb	1998
Transgenic mouse models of hereditary pancreatitis – pathophysiology	L	C.D. Ullrich 2nd	1999
Transgenic models	L	J. Jänne	2000
Gene targeting	L	J. Brüning	2000
Transgenic models for studying endocrine tumors of the pancreas	L	G. Rindi	2000
Molecular genetics of pancreatic cancer	L	N. Lemoine	2000
SPINK 1 mutations in chronic pancreatitis	L	H. Witt	2001
Gene therapy for pancreatic cancer – gene correction by sst 2	L	L. Buscail	2001
Gene therapy for pancreatic cancer – intratumoral targeted chemotherapy	L	M. Löhr	2001
Familial pancreatic cancer, hereditary pancreatitis	S	Toulouse, EUROPAC	2001
What can genetics tell us about the pathophysiology of chronic pancreatitis?	L	D. Whitcomb	2003
New genetic aspects of cystic fibrosis	L	J.M. Rommens	1990
The adult cystic fibrosis patient: Problems and therapeutic advances	L	G. Mastella	1994
Cystic fibrosis and the pancreas	L	S. Nousia-Arvanitakis	1998
Is idiopathic chronic pancreatitis cystic fibrosis?	L	J.A. Cohn	1999

two lectures by D. Whitcomb, one of the pioneers in the field, in 1998 and 2003. Cystic fibrosis is another example of genetically determined pancreatic involvement. Molecular analysis of genes in pancreatic diseases began in the 1990s. In three lectures (J. Rommens, 1990; G. Mastella, 1994; J. Cohn, 1999) the genetic background of cystic fibrosis was discussed, and also whether idiopathic chronic pancreatitis might have a link to cystic fibrosis (J. Cohn, 1999). SPINK 1 mutations were described in chronic pancreatitis (H. Witt, 2001). J.C. Dagorn investigated the gene regulation of pancreatic enzymes in pancreatitis (1990).

The genetics of pancreatic cancer are of special interest. Already in 1991, F. Mitelman reported on the potential value of chromosome investigations in pancreatic cancer. Our present knowledge concerning the molecular genetics of pancreatic cancer was presented by N. Lemoine in Kiel (2000). As regards possible gene therapy for pancreatic cancer, L. Buscail reported in 2001 on gene correction by sst 2 and M. Löhr (2001) on gene therapy via intratumoral targeted chemotherapy.

The EUROPAC collects data on the hereditary background of pancreatitis and pancreatic cancer in Europe in the frame of the EPC. The increasing importance of this field of genetic studies for the EPC is documented by a 1-day symposium in connection with the 37th meeting of the EPC in Graz (5th International Symposium on Inherited Diseases of the Pancreas, 9 July, 2005).

The Scientific Sessions of the EPC

The central part of the meetings without any doubt are the scientific sessions with either oral or poster presentation of new results by the members of the EPC. From 1971 to 2004, 4,837 abstracts were accepted and printed. They were presented in oral sessions (usually 25 per meeting) and also since 1977 in poster sessions (the majority). In table 15, there is a summary beginning in 1971 (the year in which the EPC meetings became uniform) until 2004. We have tried to classify the papers into three categories.

(1) Basic: Work on the physiology, biochemistry and structure of the normal pancreas, i.e. enzymes, electrolytes, hormones, secretion, neurohormonal control, enzyme synthesis, cell biology with receptors, intracellular events, stimulus-secretion coupling, and calcium signaling.

(2) Pathophysiological: Studies which are concerned with the diseased pancreas using the methods of basic research: morphology and pathophysiology of acute and chronic pancreatitis and pancreatic cancer, pathological structures, etiological agents like alcohol and their action, experimental pancreatitis, work with cancer cell lines, and function of the diseased pancreas in humans.

(3) Clinical: Clinical picture of acute and chronic pancreatitis, pancreatic carcinoma, natural history of these diseases, diagnostics, epidemiology, conservative and surgical approaches.

Table 15. The number of scientific presentations at the meetings of the EPC from 1971 to 2004

	1971 Brussels	1973 Gothenburg	1974 Dundee	1975 Toulouse	1976 Oslo	1977 Dublin	1978 Zürich	1979 Copenhagen
Basic	22	40	25	46	36	37	42	49
Pathophysiological	26	30	20	28	24	49	32	42
Clinical	16	20	24	31	23	55	24	48
Total	64	90	69	105	83	141	98	139
Basic, %	34	44	36	43	43	26	42	34
Basic + pathophysiological, %	75	77	62	70	72	60	75	64

	1981 Krakow	1982 Essen	1983 Verona	1984 Cascais	1985 Manchester	1986 Nijmegen	1987 Marseilles	1988 Budapest
Basic	36	51	54	41	67	47	51	48
Pathophysiological	51	48	33	33	46	58	55	51
Clinical	35	50	44	49	37	46	45	51
Total	122	149	131	123	150	151	151	150
Basic, %	29	34	41	33	44	31	33	32
Basic + pathophysiological, %	71	66	66	61	75	69	70	66

	1989 Glasgow	1990 Basel	1991 Lund	1992 Ulm	1993 Paris	1994 Bologna	1995 Barcelona	1996 Mannheim
Basic	43	55	45	31	35	35	30	33
Pathophysiological	66	55	49	62	68	67	58	90
Clinical	67	57	56	63	44	78	72	54
Total	176	167	150	156	147	180	160	177
Basic, %	25	32	30	21	23	19	18	18
Basic + pathophysiological, %	62	65	62		70	56	55	69

	1997 London	1998 Thessaloniki	1999 Lüneburg	2000 Kiel	2001 Toulouse	2002 Heidelberg	2003 Liverpool	2004 Padova
Basic	38	21	24	16	22	22	13	20
Pathophysiological	94	62	73	72	73	140	61	80
Clinical	93	91	53	64	64	167	96	98
Total	225	174	150	152	159	331	170	198
Basic, %	16	12	16	10	13	6	7	10
Basic + pathophysiological, %	58	47	64	58	59	49	43	49

It was the rule of the EPC that about 60% of the papers should deal with basic science and pathophysiology and around 40% with clinical work. Table 14 demonstrates that this was the case over many years. On average, in the years until 1985 the percentage of papers dedicated to pure basic research was around 30–40% and from 1986 to 1993 around 25–30%; slowly this percentage declined to around 15–20%. Since 2000 basic topics are found only in 6–10%. Concomitantly the number of sessions, which were dedicated to basic topics such as enzymes, stimulus-secretion coupling, neurohormonal control of secretion, and receptors shrunk from as many as 5 or more in the early years to only 1 or 2 from the middle of the 1990s on. On the other hand, the papers with topics on pathology and pathophysiology were always about 25–35%. They increased in number from the 1990s and partly compensated for the decline in papers on basic science. Looking at the content, a specific increase in papers concerned with problems of carcinogenesis can be observed since the mid 1990s.

The percentage of clinical papers was low in the early years with 25–30%. Over time they slowly increased in number, in the last years since 1998 they have been approaching 40–50%.

In table 16, we show the absolute figures of abstracts dealing with basic science, pathophysiology or pure clinical work. We must look at these figures in conjunction with those in table 14. Basic science contributions had been in the range of 40–60 per meeting over many years until 1991; then the number declined to 30–40 per meeting till 1997, after that it went down to only 13–22 per meeting. At the same time the number of pure clinical papers increased to around 90 per meeting. In 2002, the figures were especially high (167) due to the joint meeting of EPC and IAP in Heidelberg.

Abstracts dealing with the pathophysiology of pancreatic diseases are very important in the sense that they reflect the applied effect of basic science on the clinical laboratories. This is one of the goals of the EPC. The number of abstracts in this category was stable around 30–50 per meeting until 1985, then it rose slowly to 60–70 and since 1995 up to 90. As shown in table 17, this increase is mainly due to work with carcinoma cell lines and not with 'classical' pathophysiology. The profile of interest in the diseases of the pancreas has changed over time (table 17).

Since 1981, acute pancreatitis was the issue of an increasing number of papers, whereas interest in chronic pancreatitis has decreased. This disease was a main topic of clinical research in the 1970s. One reason for the preference for acute pancreatitis might be the easier research with experimental models, which are still lacking in chronic pancreatitis. This also holds true in the field of pancreatic carcinoma. The work with cancer cell lines has increased greatly from the beginning of the 1980s. From 1981 to 1985, there were only 19 papers on experimental carcinoma, while from 1996 to 2000 there were 96.

On the Problem of Declining Contributions to Basic Science

Without doubt the phenomenon of decreasing contributions from basic scientists is a very severe problem. It is the contrary of the ideas of the founding era to bring basic scientists and clinicians together to create mutual stimulation of the work, and also to encourage friendship which grows in the familiar atmosphere of a relatively small scientific society (compared to others). Obviously this held true in the first 30 years of the Club, but now it seems to be changing.

What could be the reasons for this development? We would like to list a few ideas.

Table 16. Absolute number of abstracts dealing with basic science, pathophysiology or pure clinical work

	1971–1975	1976–1979 (4 years)	1981–1985	1986–1990	1991–1995	1996–2000	2001–2004 (4 years)
Basic	133	164	249	244	176	132	77
Pathophysiology	104	147	211	283	304	391	354
Clinical	91	150	215	303	313	355	425

Table 17. Number of abstracts on acute and chronic pancreatitis and carcinoma cell lines

	1981–1985	1986–1990	1991–1995	1996–2000	2001–2004
Acute pancreatitis	52	155	218	283	158
Chronic pancreatitis	112	55	87	139	129
Carcinoma	59	92	189	202	179

(1) In the last years a number of laboratories, also clinical-experimental ones, with pancreatic research, no longer participated because of retirement or waning interest in the EPC of that particular group. Examples are the groups of Jean Christophe in Brussels, of Henri Sarles in Marseilles, J.J. de Pont in Nijmegen, Irene Schulz in Homburg, Werner Creutzfeldt in Göttingen and Harald Goebell in Essen. Their activities have only partially been replaced by followers. New young working groups in particular should, therefore, be invited and encouraged to attend the meetings. (2) The officers of the Club are mostly clinicians. In the 40 years of the Club we had only 9 basic scientists as Presidents (J. Christophe in 1971, S.J. Konturek in 1981, M. Case in 1985, J.J. de Pont in 1986, C. Rozé in 1993, G.E. Mann in 1997, N. Vaysse in 2001, O.H. Petersen in 2003 and T. Grieshaber in 2005). This was one of the reasons why the new statutes mandate a basic scientist President for every other year. (3) The structure of the meetings does not attract basic scientists. Maybe some parallel sessions with basic papers would give more space to them for discussions with colleagues. To have in 2.5 days only one session with these topics is not attractive. In the first 20–30 years we had at least 4–6 sessions dedicated to basic contributions. (4) Big meetings like the joint ones of EPC and IAP are dominated by clinicians, mainly also surgeons, and are not attractive for basic scientists. The presidents of those meetings must be especially careful to counteract the trend of too many clinical sessions with the character of postgraduate train-

Table 18. Lectures given at the Young Researchers Corner

1993	Paris	Cultured cell, receptors, cell pathing, calcium signaling (Clemente, Estival, Williams, Petersen)
1994	Bologna	Methodology for the study of pancreatic receptors (de Weerth, Fourmy, Jensen, Buscail, Susini)
1995	Barcelona	Methodology for the study of genetic alterations in pancreatic cancer (Löhr, Fernandez, Lemoine, Peinado)
1996	Mannheim	Methodology in pancreatic physiology (Schmidt, Holst, Teyssen, Niebergall-Roth, Gullo)
1997	London	Signal transduction in islet and exocrine cells: Overview of methodology (Pedley, Elliott, Willems, Dunne, Persaud)
1998	Thessaloniki	Models of experimental pancreatitis and relevance to human disease (Lerch, Mössner, Vollmar, Ward, Beglinger)
1999	Lüneburg	Clinical epidemiology and biostatistics for the pancreatologists (Lowenfels, Bueno-de Mesquita)
2000	Kiel	Researchers think tank: Pancreatic cancer cells, genetics of cancer, pancreatic stellate cells (Klöppel, Schmid, Real, Lemoine, Wagner, Kalthoff, Pinzani, Wilson, Sjöholm)
2001	Toulouse	Genomic and post-genomic developments in biomedical sciences (Gress, Ferec, Prats, Pramanik)
2002	Heidelberg	Genetics, microdissection, proteomics, cell culture, transcriptomics (Hoheisel, Kleef, Scarpa, Costello, Siech, Löhr)
2003	Liverpool	Real time imaging of the pancreas: Confocal and 2-photon microscopy, electrophysiology, uncaging techniques (Tepikin, Maruyama, Ashby, Lerch)
2004	Padova	New biotechnologies in the diagnostic and therapeutic approach to pancreatic diseases: Use of microarrays, gene therapy (Lanfranchi, Gress, Sangro, Maruyama)

ing. (5) The sponsoring by pharmaceutical companies might be an additional push towards too many clinical topics and should be observed. (6) The social side of the meetings must be of special interest to the organizers because in such a small society this can create the contacts and friendship which are also needed for research cooperation.

The authors think that one of the positive results of their work on the history of the EPC is to draw attention to these problems. They suggest that a small working group of representative EPC experts should be created for further analysis of the problem and for planning counteractions.

One of the strategies to reverse these trends has already been introduced, the Young Researchers Corner.

The Young Researchers Corner

In 1993, Claude Rozé started a new program: the Young Researchers Corner. The idea was to attract young people interested in learning methods of basic research in the field of the pancreas. Since then this small program has run successfully at all meetings. Top experts in their field were invited to give lectures (table 18).

What Stood the Test of Time?

One of us (Werner Creutzfeldt), being one the 9 founding members in 1965, had been asked to give a lecture at the 32nd EPC meeting in Lüneburg in 1999 with this title. Based on the material concerning the scientific profile of the meetings of the Club we would like to answer this question. The EPC meetings summarized our knowledge at the time in a great number of state-of-the-art and invited lectures and symposia of experts. The meetings were also accepted as platforms for the presentation of current research and of new results with an immense number of published abstracts. All topics have been investigated. So it is justified to put the question of what remains.

Physiology, Biochemistry, Cell Biology (table 19)

The pancreas obviously attracted the interest of a significant number of excellent basic researchers and the EPC can be glad that they regarded this Club as a panel to present their data.

The pancreatic acinar cell with its ability to synthesize large amounts of proteins, the sorting and package of these proteins and transport in zymogen granules to the membrane seems to be ideal to study these basic biological processes. Already in the 1950s, George E. Palade and his group analyzed the morphological steps in this process (Nobel Prize in 1974). The analysis of gastrointestinal hormones (secretin, cholecystokinin-pancreozymin, gastrin, and others like bombesin or vasointestinal peptide), the studies of their receptors, and the interplay with the neural system resulted in fascinating results. The neurohormonal control of secretion, therefore, was a big issue at many EPC meetings. The intracellular events which follow this stimulation in the acinar and in the ductal cells (stimulus-secretion coupling, intracellular signaling, es-

Table 19. Physiology, biochemistry, cell biology of the pancreas: What stood the test of time?

Gastrointestinal hormones and pancreas	yes
Nerves and pancreatic stimulation	yes
Neurohormonal control of secretion	yes
Receptors and second messengers	yes
Protein synthesis, transport, secretion	yes
Intracellular signaling, stimulus-secretion coupling, role of calcium	yes
Islet cell-acinar interrelationship	yes
Entero-insular axis (incretins)	yes
Genetic basis of inherited pancreatic disorders	yes

Table 20. Experimental work on pancreatic disease: What stood the test of time?

Pathogenesis of pancreatitis and cancer	
Enzyme activation (proteases, lipases)	yes
Explanation of the mechanisms	no
Analysis of pathophysiology of acute pancreatitis	yes
Infected necrosis as major risk factor for mortality	yes
Feedback control of pancreatic secretion by intraduodenal trypsin in man	no
Pancreatic stone protein	no
Molecular and cell biology of pancreatic cancer	yes
Miscellaneous	
Attempts to attract diabetologists (the pancreas: one organ or two?)	no
The informality of the EPC	?
To promote the exchange of ideas and the friendship between basic and clinical scientists in Europe	yes

pecially the role of calcium) are even today a matter of research with model character. Also, the studies of interactions between the gut and the islet cells (enteroinsular axis) and of islet cells and the acinar cells have yielded many insights. All these results stood the test of time. Many of the classical studies on hormonal and nerval regulation of pancreatic secretion both in animals and in humans have been carried out by clinical investigators in clinical laboratories oriented to basic research.

Pathogenesis of Pancreatitis and of Pancreatic Cancer (table 20)

The studies on activation of enzymes in the pancreas have shown that these processes, especially the activation of trypsinogen and other proenzymes, play a decisive role in the pathogenesis of acute pancreatitis. Also, the place of lysosomes in this context is interesting. But we have no stringent explanation yet despite extensive experimental work of what mechanism really sets off the starting process of acute pancreatitis.

Good progress has been made with the explanation of the pathophysiology of pancreatic inflammation and its consequences for the whole organism. The key role of infection of the pancreas in the course of acute pancreatitis with respect to morbidity and mortality has been better defined. This knowledge has contributed significantly to a better and consistent treatment of the patients and a better survival chance. We have no explanation yet of which steps lead to the evolution of chronic pancreatitis with its variations (noncalcifying, calcifying). The role of alcohol intake and action is still unclear. The possible existence of a calcium binding PSP and its diminished secretion in chronic pancreatitis could not be proved and did not stand the test of time. The finding that the concentration of trypsin in the duodenum inhibits the secretion of CCK (feedback control) in animals gave hope for a therapeutic effect of pancreatic enzymes in humans with severe pancreatic pain in chronic pancreatitis. However, this could not been confirmed in patients. Finally, the studies of molecular and cell biology and the corresponding gene defects of pancreatic cancer obviously open new therapeutic perspectives. But this field has only just been opened.

Methods for Diagnosis of Pancreatic Diseases (table 21)

Since the 1950s, it has been one of the aims to develop tests for the function of the exocrine pancreas. Knowledge increased that in chronic pancreatitis as consequence of the destruction of the tissue a progressive diminution of the function occurs. The secretion of enzymes and of bicarbonate decreases, leading eventually to maldigestion of all nutrients. Test meals with an estimation of the enzyme concentration in duodenal juice (Lundh test) were not reliable enough and also the idea that the stimulation of the pancreas results in a different elevation of amylase/lipase in the blood according to the remaining functional tissue leads to erratic results (evocative tests). The development of a functional test was accomplished by the use of secretin (fluid and bicarbonate) and pancreozymin-cholecystokinin/cerulein (enzymes) and analysis of the duodenal/pancreatic juice. The members of the EPC cooperated closely in the standardization of this test, which was time-consuming, but sensitive and reproducible, the gold standard in scientific studies. For practical purposes, Ammann developed a method for the estimation of chymotrypsin in feces (nowadays replaced by elastase) as a

Table 21. Methods for diagnosis of pancreatic diseases: What stood the test of time?

Pancreatic function tests	
Evocative tests	no
Test meal	no
Secretin-CCK (cerulein) test	yes
Enzymes in feces	yes
Tubeless absorption tests (PABA and pancreolauryl tests)	yes
Amino acid consumption test	no
Imaging methods	
Angiography	no
Tomography and pneumoperitoneum	no
^{75}Se scintigraphy	no
Endoscopic retrograde pancreatography (ERP)	yes
Computer tomography (CT)	yes
Ultrasonography	yes
Endoscopic ultrasonography	yes
Magnetic resonance imaging (MR)	yes
MR cholangiopancreatography (MRCP)	yes
Positron emission tomography (PET)	yes
Somatostatin receptor scintigraphy for endocrine tumor localization	yes

Table 22. Treatment of acute pancreatitis: What stood the test of time?

1 Enzyme inhibitors	
Aprotinin (Trasylol) 1960–1978	no
Gabexate mesilate (Foy) 1980–1990	no
2 Inhibitors of enzyme secretion	
Calcitonin	no
Glucagon	no
Somatostatin	no
Octreotide	no
3 Inhibition of inflammatory mediators	
Lexipafant (PAF antagonist), 1997	no
Antioxidant, sodium selenite, 1997	no
4 Intensive care	
Systematic basic and problem-oriented therapy	yes
Prognostic scores	yes
Visualization of necrotic areas in the pancreas (contrast-enhanced dynamic CT)	yes
5 Surgical intervention	
Total pancreatectomy	no
Early operation	no
Early ERCP and papillotomy without obstructive jaundice	no
Necrosectomy, drainage	yes

simple clinical test, ideal for the follow-up of patients; it is, however, less sensitive and quantitative than the secretin-CCK test. Tubeless absorption tests with the splitting of orally applied nonabsorbable esters (PABA = N-benzoyl-*L*-tyrosyl-para-aminobenzoic acid) by trypsin and of pancreolauryl-fluorescein by pseudocholesterolesterase (pankreolauryl test) and the respective increase of the digestion products in blood in correlation to the normal or diminished amount of trypsin or esterases in the duodenum are elegant, but have not found broad distribution. Finally, the use of the consumption of amino acids in the pancreas as a marker test for the synthetic capacity of the gland did not prove to be reproducible.

Imaging of the pancreas has shown great progress since the 1980s. Evolving from the classical radiology, angiography was developed for the detection of pancreatic cancer, and also scintigraphy of the pancreas with ^{75}Se-tagged methionine. They were soon abandoned when the ERP set standards for the imaging of the duct system. The external ultrasound investigation and the newer endoscopic endosonography opened new possibilities for the daily practice. Computer tomography, also with the dynamic contrast-enhanced technique for the detection of necrotic areas in the inflamed pancreas, magnetic resonance and MRCP set absolute new fascinating possibilities for the imaging of the pancreas and its ducts. Nevertheless, the early diagnosis of pancreatic carcinoma is still difficult. In some cases the PET may detect early small tumors especially when combined with CT investigation (PET-CT). A very elegant method for the detection of hormone-producing endocrine tumors of the pancreas and the duodenum was found through the use of tagged somatostatin (octreotide) which binds to the somatostatin receptors on the hormone-producing tumors and their metastases.

Treatment of Acute Pancreatitis (table 22)

To increase the chances of survival in patients with acute pancreatitis has been the goal for gastroenterologists and surgeons over the last century. The theories changed from being absolutely conservative ('don't touch the inflamed gland') to very aggressive approaches like total pancreatectomy. It is now generally accepted that the conservative treatment should be first in line. Results have much improved with the introduction of intensive care and systematic basic treatment, fluid, pain treatment and close supervision, in order to identify complications early and to start additional problem-oriented treatment. The development of prognostic scores sharpened the vigilance. In contrast, the search so far for specific means to

Table 23. Treatment of chronic pancreatitis and cancer: What stood the test of time?

Treatment of chronic pancreatitis	
Pancreatic oral enzyme preparation in maldigestion	yes
Oral enzymes against pain	no
Endoscopic papillotomy plus lithotripsy, stenting	yes
Drainage procedures	yes
Partial pancreatic resection	yes
Duodenum-preserving resection of pancreatic head	yes
Treatment of pancreatic carcinoma	
Early surgery	yes
Chemotherapy	no
Radiotherapy	no

positively influence the course of the disease has failed (enzyme inhibitors, inhibitors of pancreatic secretion such as glucagon, calcitonin, somatostatin). Multicenter trials (also within the framework of the EPC) laid the ground for these experiences. Surgical intervention was also critically evaluated. Total pancreatectomy was abandoned as well as early intervention. Drainage procedures, especially of the infected necrosis, together with necrosectomy and antibiotics in well-planned time frames have found their place and have increased the chances of the patients. ERCP is not indicated in idiopathic acute pancreatitis. In gallstone pancreatitis the performance of ERCP has increased the diagnostic certainty. However, early ERCP with papillotomy in biliary pancreatitis cases without obstructive jaundice is not justified. In three prospective studies (Fan, Neoptolemos, Fölsch) there was no benefit regarding the mortality and in two studies also regarding the complications of biliary pancreatitis.

Treatment of Chronic Pancreatitis and Carcinoma (table 23)

Maldigestion is one of the leading symptoms of advanced chronic pancreatitis due to the lack of pancreatic enzymes in the gut, thus leading to steatorrhea and weight loss. The enzyme deficiency can be compensated for by oral replacement of enzymes. Enzymes easing the pancreatic pain, based on the idea of a feedback inhibition of CCK-stimulated pancreatic secretion by intraluminal proteases, have failed. The endoscopic interventional methods with stenting and lithotripsy have given at least temporary relief. Surgical drainage procedures and partial pancreatectomy have proved to be beneficial. New methods of resection of the pancreatic head with preservation of the duodenum (Beger resection) have brought progress in comparison with the classical Whipple procedure.

The new imaging methods have increased the chances for earlier detection of the developing tumor. So early surgery has better chances than before. Trials with chemotherapy and radiation on the other hand have ultimately not yet found a beneficial outcome.

Conclusion

Looking back on 40 years of the EPC and of pancreatic research we are proud that the result is positive. When the 9 founders met in 1965, they had the vision that the existence of a forum of investigators with a common interest in the pancreas would promote both, basic and clinical research.

The founders of the Club relied upon the interacting forces of friendship in informal surroundings. This turned out to be true. Numerous contacts developed. Many young researchers went to other laboratories, got new ideas with the help of the EPC and multicenter studies were encouraged. Especially the idea that basic research (physiology, biochemistry, molecular biology, genetics) has much to contribute beyond the mere interest in biological mechanisms for the benefit of a better life for patients with diseases of the pancreas proved to be positive. On the other hand, the analysis of the scientific sessions of the EPC revealed that in the last 10 years the number of contributions from basic scientists has markedly decreased. This is a phenomenon which is in contrast to the ideas of the founders and must be seriously counteracted by the officers of the EPC who are responsible for the future of the EPC.

At the end of our work about the history of the EPC we would like to say that in 40 years this scientific society has stood the test of time and will also stand it in the future.

Acknowledgments

We thank Mrs. Rita Shinkle for checking the linguistic quality of the manuscript and Professor Maynard Case and Professor Markus Lerch for their critical comments, which helped to make the manuscript more precise and readable.

Reference

1 Andren-Sandberg A, Johnson C: A quantitative analysis of European pancreatic research as reflected by abstracts from the annual European Pancreatic Club meetings 1982–1997 (abstract 167). Digestion 1998;59:262.

Pancreatology

Pancreatology 2005;5(suppl 1):35–102
DOI: 10.1159/000086077

Published online: June 3, 2005

37th European Pancreatic Club (EPC) Meeting

Abstracts

July 6–8, 2005,
Graz, Austria

Guest Editor
Thomas Griesbacher, Graz

Contents

KARGER

Basel · Freiburg · Paris · London · New York ·
Bangalore · Bangkok · Singapore · Tokyo · Sydney

Basic Sciences

1

A Novel Method for Gene Transfer to Isolated Pancreatic Ducts

M. Kovacs[1,3,4], *Z. Rakonczay Jr.*[2,1], *B. Ordog*[3], *T. Takács*[1], *J. Lonovics*[1], *A. Varro*[4], *A. Toth*[4], *J.G. Papp*[4], *M.A. Gray*[2], *B.E. Argent*[2], *Z. Boldogkoi*[3], *P. Hegyi*[1,2]

[1]First Department of Medicine Faculty of Medicine, University of Szeged, Hungary; [2]School of Cell & Molecular Biosciences, University Medical School, Newcastle upon Tyne, UK; [3]Department of Biology, Faculty of Medicine, University of Szeged, Hungary, [4]Department of Pharmacology and Pharmacotherapy, Faculty of Medicine, Division of Cardiovascular Pharmacology, Hungarian Academy of Sciences, University of Szeged, Hungary

Background: Several types of viral vectors are currently in use for gene transfer, but there is no available method to transfect intact pancreatic ducts. Viral invasion of cells may lead to cytotoxicity, which may question the validity of any observations. Our aim was to establish a model system for transferring genes into the pancreatic duct cells, which did not lead to cell damage.

Methods: The non-virulent Ka-RREp0lacgfp (KEG) genetically modified strain of pseudorabies virus (PRV) containing the gene for GFP was used in this study. Small intra/interlobular ducts were isolated from the pancreas of guinea pigs. Ducts were incubated in McCoy's based culture medium containing KEG virus at four different titers (10^7, 10^8, 10^9 and 10^{10} plaque forming units/ml) for 6 hours. The rate of HCO_3^- secretion was determined as described previously (Hegyi et al. Am J Physiol Cell Physiol 2003;285:C268–C276). Viral structural proteins were visualized by immunohistochemistry. Native GFP expression and immunofluorescence signals were recorded by a confocal laser scanning microscope.

Results: We observed that KEG virus infected practically all accessible epithelial cells within the duct when used at a titer of 10^{10} pfu/ml after 24 hours as judged by the appearance of GFP. Importantly, we did not observe any cytotoxic effects of KEG and could not detect viral antigens on the cell surface, indicating the lack of viral replication. KEG did not affect ductal HCO_3^- secretion at any of the titers tested.

Conclusions: The high efficiency of PRV infection in the pancreatic ductal epithelium may open the possibility for gene transfer and gene therapy of the duct cells using non-replicating PRV variants.

This work was supported by The Wellcome Trust and OTKA.

2

The Effects of Substance P on HCO_3^- Transport in Guinea Pig Microperfused Pancreatic Ducts

P. Hegyi[1], *Z. Rakonczay Jr.*[2,1], *T. Takács*[1], *J.G. Papp*[3], *J. Lonovics*[1], *A. Toth*[3], *A. Varro*[3], *M.A. Gray*[2], *B.E. Argent*[2]

[1]First Department of Medicine, [3]Department of Pharmacology and Pharmacotherapy, Division of Cardiovascular Pharmacology, Hungarian Academy of Sciences, Faculty of Medicine, University of Szeged, Hungary; [2]Institute for Cell & Molecular Biosciences, University Medical School, Newcastle upon Tyne, UK

Background: We have previously shown using sealed, non-perfused, ducts that Substance P (SP) inhibits HCO_3^- secretion by inhibiting Cl^- dependent HCO_3^- efflux on the luminal membrane of the duct cell (Hegyi et al. Am J Physiol Cell Physiol 2003;285:C268–C276). However, in that study we had no direct evidence that SP affected a luminal anion exchanger. To address this issue we examined the effects of luminal H_2DIDS on the inhibitory effect of SP in microperfused ducts.

Methods: Small intra/interlobular pancreatic ducts were isolated from guinea pigs. We microperfused the ducts allowing direct access to the luminal membrane of the duct cell. The rate of HCO_3^- secretion was determined by measuring the initial rate of intracellular acidification (using BCECF) following sudden block of basolateral $NaHCO_3$ cotransporters and Na^+/H^+ exchangers with H_2DIDS (500 μM) and amiloride (200 μM) respectively. The buffering capacity of duct cells was estimated and the rate of transmembrane H^+ flux, $J(H^+)$, was calculated. Since H^+ and HCO_3^- will largely be derived from H_2CO_3, we have assumed that $J(H^+)$ is equivalent to $J(HCO_3)$. All the experiments were performed in HCO_3^--buffered Ringer at 37°C.

Results: Rates of HCO_3^- secretion measured using the inhibitor stop method were about 2 fold higher in microperfused ducts as compared to sealed, non-perfused, ducts. Application of luminal H_2DIDS (0.5 mM) caused intracellular pH to alkalinise and, like SP, inhibited basal and secretin-stimulated HCO_3^- secretion. SP did not inhibit secretion further when H_2DIDS was present in the lumen, suggesting that SP and H_2DIDS both inhibit the same transporter on the luminal membrane of the duct cell.

Conclusions: SP inhibits an H_2DIDS-sensitive HCO_3^- transport step at the luminal membrane of the duct cell, most likely a member of the SLC26 family anion exchanger.

This work was supported by The Wellcome Trust and OTKA.

KARGER

Fax +41 61 306 12 34
E-Mail karger@karger.ch
www.karger.com

1424–3903/05/0057–0036$22.00/0

Accessible online at:
www.karger.com/pan

3

A Physiological Role of Substance P in the Inhibitory Control of Pancreatic Ductal HCO_3^- Secretion

B. Ózsvári[1], Z. Rakonczay Jr.[2,1], L. Tiszlavicz[3], T. Takács[1], J.G. Papp[4], J. Lonovics[1], A. Toth[4], G. Racz[5], G. Varga[5], M.A. Gray[2], B.E. Argent[2], P. Hegyi[1,2], G.Z. Rácz

[1]First Department of Medicine, [3]Department of Pathology and [4]Department of Pharmacology and Pharmacotherapy, Division of Cardiovascular Pharmacology, Hungarian Academy of Sciences, Faculty of Medicine, University of Szeged, Hungary; [2]Institute for Cell & Molecular Biosciences, University Medical School, Newcastle upon Tyne, UK; [5]Molecular Oral Biology Research Group, Department of Oral Biology, Hungarian Academy of Sciences and Semmelweis University, Budapest, Hungary

Background: The inhibitory control of pancreatic ductal HCO_3^- secretion may be physiologically important in terms of limiting the hydrostatic pressure developed within the ducts and in terms of switching off pancreatic secretion after a meal. Substance P (SP) inhibits secretin-stimulated HCO_3^- secretion by modulating a Cl^--dependent HCO_3^- efflux step at the apical membrane of the duct cell (Hegyi et al. Am J Physiol Cell Physiol 2003;285:C268–C276). In the present study we have sought to localise SP in the guinea-pig pancreas and to identify the intracellular signalling pathway utilised by SP.

Methods: Small intra/interlobular pancreatic ducts were isolated from guinea pigs. The rate of HCO_3^- secretion was determined from intracellular pH measurements as previously described (Hegyi et al., 2003). Western blot analysis was used to identify PKC isoforms expressed in the isolated ducts and immunohistochemistry to localize SP in the pancreas.

Results: Our results show that SP is present in periductal nerves within the guinea-pig pancreas and that protein kinase C (PKC) mediates the effect of SP. Secretin (10 nM) stimulated HCO_3^- secretion by sealed, non-perfused, ducts about 3 fold and this effect was totally inhibited by SP (20 nM). Phorbol 12,13-dibutyrate (PDBu; 100 nM), an activator of PKC, reduced basal HCO_3^- secretion by about 40%, and totally blocked secretin-stimulated secretion. In addition, bisindolylmaleimide I (1 nM to 1 μM), an inhibitor of PKC, relieved the inhibitory effect of SP on secretin-stimulated HCO_3^- secretion. Western blot analysis revealed that guinea pig pancreatic ducts express the $-\alpha$, $-\beta I$, $-\delta$, $-\varepsilon$, $-\eta$, $-\theta$, $-\zeta$ and $-\mu$ isoforms of PKC.

Conclusions: Taken together, our results indicate that SP reduces HCO_3^- secretion in guinea pig ducts via activation of PKC, which inhibits a luminal Cl^-/HCO_3^- exchanger (most likely a member of the SLC26 family).

This work was supported by The Wellcome Trust and OTKA.

4

Dual Age-Dependent Effect of Ghrelin Administration on the Pancreatic Growth in Young Rats and its Relation to IGF-1 Release

A. Dembiński[1], Z. Warzecha[1], P. Ceranowicz[1], W. Bielanski[1], M. Dembiński[1], W.W. Pawlik[1], P.C. Konturek[2], A. Kuwahara[3], I. Kato[4]

[1]Department of Physiology, Jagiellonian University Medical College, Krakow, Poland; [2]Department of Internal Medicine I, University of Erlangen-Nuremberg, Erlangen, Germany; [3]Institute for Environmental Sciences, University of Shizuoka, Japan, [4]Yanaihara Institute Inc., Shizuoka, Japan

Background: Ghrelin is a circulating growth hormone-releasing peptide primary isolated from the human and rat stomach. Ghrelin stimulates the appetite and fat deposition in adult rats and humans. The aim of study was to investigate the effect of ghrelin on pancreatic growth in suckling, weaned and peripubertal seven-week-old rats.

Methods: Rats were treated with saline or ghrelin (4, 8 or 16 nmol/kg/dose) intraperitoneally twice a day: suckling rats were treated for 7 or 14 days starting from the first postnatal day, three-week-old weaned rats were treated for 1 or 5 days, seven-week-old rats were treated for 4 days.

Results: Treatment with ghrelin did not affect animal weight in suckling or weaned rats, whereas in young seven-week-old rats, ghrelin caused a significant increase in body weight. Ghrelin decreased food intake in weaned rats, whereas in seven-week-old rats, food intake was enhanced. In suckling rats, ghrelin decreased the pancreatic weight, pancreatic amylase content, DNA synthesis and DNA content. In contrast, ghrelin in weaned or young seven-week-old rats increased pancreatic weight, DNA synthesis, DNA content and amylase content. Pancreatic blood flow was not affected by ghrelin in any group of rats tested. Ghrelin increased serum level of growth hormone in all rats. This effect was weak in suckling rats, higher in weaned and the highest in seven-week-old animals. Ghrelin did not affect serum level of IGF-1 in suckling rats. In weaned and in seven-week-old rats, treatment with ghrelin caused increase in serum level of IGF-1, whereas in suckling rats ghrelin did not affect serum level of IGF-1.

Conclusions: Ghrelin reduced pancreatic growth in suckling rats, whereas in weaned and young seven-week-old animals, treatment with ghrelin increased pancreatic growth. This biphasic effect of ghrelin in young animals on pancreatic growth seems to be related to age-dependent changes of the release of anabolic IGF-1.

5

Evidence for a Direct and Functional Interaction between the Human CCK2 Receptor and RGS2

I. Langer, I. Tikhonova, S. Vatinel, A. Ferrand, F. Lopez, J.P. Estève, L. Moroder, C. Boulegue, D. Fourmy

INSERM U531, Laboratoire de Biologie et Pathologies Digestives, TSA 50032 CHU Rangueil Bat L3, Toulouse, France

Introduction: Regulators of G protein signalling (RGS proteins) are a family of diverse, multifunctional proteins that share a conserved 120 amino acid domain (RGS box). RGS box binds directly to activated Gα subunits and acts as GTPase-activating proteins (GAPs) to attenuate and/or modulate G Protein-Coupled Receptor (GPCR) mediated signalling. The mechanisms by which individual RGS proteins desensitize pathways activated by particular GPCRs remain to be elucidated. We investigated the molecular basis for targeting individual RGS proteins to type-2 cholecystokinin/gastrin receptor (CCK2R) which is the predominant cholecystokinin receptor in the human pancreas.

Methods: We constructed amino-terminally truncated RGS2, overexpressed them in COS-7 cells and evaluated their inhibitory effect on CCK2R-mediated inositol phosphate accumulation. We also performed pull down and molecular modelling experiments.

Results: We found that removal of the 80 amino acids preceding the RGS box completely abolishes RGS2 activity but that activity was restored by adding the sequence comprised between residues 54 and 80 of RGS2. The same approach was used to identify potential CCK2R domains involved in direct interaction with RGS2: we found that removal of a 10 amino acids sequence (429–439) in the carboxyl-terminus tail of CCK2R abolishes the inhibitory effect of RGS2. Pull down experiments confirmed that RGS2 and CCK2R interact together and that the identified sequences were directly involved. These results allowed us to build a 3D model of [RGS2.CCK2R] complex and to identify more precisely the amino acids responsible for a direct interaction between RGS2 and the CCK2R.

Conclusion: In conclusion, for the first time, we have demonstrated a direct interaction between a GPCR and an RGS, namely RGS2 and CCK2R which is the predominant cholecystokinin receptor in the human pancreas, and identified the involved peptidic sequences on both partners.

6

A Novel Signaling Pathway Coupling Secretory Activity and Gene Expression in Pancreatic β-Cells

H. Mziaut[1], M. Trajkovski[1], A. Altkruger[1], M.-S. Lee[2], H.D. Saeger[3], S. Kersting[3], M. Solimena[1]

[1]Experimental Diabetology and [3]Dept. of Surgery, 'Carl Gustav Carus' Medical School, University of Technology, Dresden, Germany; [2]Samsung Medical Center, Seoul, Korea

Introduction: An important question in diabetes is how β-cells adjust the production of new insulin secretory granules (ISGs) according to their secretory activity. Recently we demonstrated that exocytosis of ISGs is associated with the cleavage of the cytoplasmic domain of islet cell autoantigen 512 (ICA512/IA-2), a receptor tyrosine phosphatase-like protein of the ISG membrane. The resulting ICA512 cleaved cytosolic fragment (ICA512-CCF) is targeted to the nucleus, where it up-regulates insulin gene expression (Trajkovski et al. J Cell Biol 2004;167:1063–1074).

Methods: Using insulinoma INS-1 cells and pancreatic islets isolated from ICA512 KO mice and control littermates as model systems for molecular cell biological analyses, we investigated how ICA512-CCF regulates gene expression.

Results: We demonstrate that ICA512-CCF regulates the expression of insulin and that of other genes required for SG assembly, including ICA512 itself, through the STAT pathway. STATs are transcription factors, which are activated by cytokines and growth factors, and which up-regulate insulin gene expression as well as β-cell proliferation. Specifically, we show that knockdown of STAT5b expression by RNA-interference decreases ICA512 levels. Conversely, overexpression of ICA512-CCF increases the levels of nuclear STAT5b, mainly due to the accumulation of phosphorylated STAT5. Co-immunoprecipitation assays showed that ICA512-CCF and STAT5b are part of a complex, while electrophoretic mobility shift assays indicated that ICA512-CCF increases the binding of STAT5 to its own recognition element in the insulin 1 gene promoter. Finally, chromatin co-immunoprecipitation assays demonstrated that ICA512-CCF is itself associated with the STAT5 binding element in the insulin 1 gene promoter, conceivably via its association with the STA5b.

Conclusions: We have discovered a novel feedback pathway, whereby ICA512 directly couples regulated exocytosis of ISGs with regulation of gene expression of β-cells via STATs. These findings may provide insight for elucidating the pathogenesis of diabetes and the development of novel treatments for its therapy.

7

Transcriptome Analysis of Human Hepatic and Pancreatic Stellate Cells: Organ-Specific Variation of a Common Transcriptional Phenotype

M. Buchholz[1], H.A. Kestler[1,3], K. Holzmann[1], V. Ellenrieder[1], W. Schneiderhan[2], M. Siech[4], G. Adler[1], M.G. Bachem[2], T.M. Gress[1]

[1]Abteilung Innere Medizin I, and [2]Abt. Klinische Chemie, Universitätsklinikum Ulm; [3]Stiftungsdozentur Bioinformatik, Universität Ulm; [4]Abt. Allgemein- Visceral- und Gefäßchirurgie, Ostalb-Klinikum Aalen, Germany

Introduction: Pancreatic stellate cells (PSC) are thought to be the primary source of the extensive fibrotic reaction which is a hallmark feature of pancreatic cancer and chronic pancreatitis. While it is well established that PSC share many morphological and functional characteristics with the more extensively studied hepatic stellate cells (HSC), the degree of similarity between the two cell types on the genetic level has remained unclear. We have analyzed the transcriptomes of HSC, PSC and normal skin fibroblasts to assess whether HSC and PSC display a common stellate cell transcriptional phenotype and if so, how it differs from that of a typical fibroblast lineage cell.

Methods: Expression profiling of short term cultures of human HSC, PSC and skin fibroblasts was performed using 23,000 feature oligonucleotide microarrays. Array data were verified using real time PCR. Functional implications of transcriptional differences were studied by mining the Gene Ontology (GO) database.

Results and discussion: The expression profiles of HSC and PSC displayed a high degree of similarity, clearly separating the stellate cells from normal skin fibroblasts. Predominantly extracellular and cell surface genes, but also signaling molecules, transcription factors and novel neural markers were concordantly expressed in both stellate cell types. Despite this high degree of similarity, distinct differences in expression patterns were observed between HSC and PSC, reflecting organ-specific variations of the common stellate cell-specific phenotype.

8

Ectopic NFAT2 Activation in Pancreatic Cancer Cells: A Novel Oncogenic Mechanism Involving Upregulation of c-myc

M. Buchholz, A. Schatz, M. Wagner, H. Mönnich, G. Adler, T.M. Gress, V. Ellenrieder

Abteilung Innere Medizin I, Universitätsklinikum Ulm, Germany

Introduction: The NFAT proteins are a family of calcium-responsive transcription factors primarily recognized for their central roles in T lymphocyte activation and cardiac valve development. Here, we demonstrate that NFAT2 is selectively overexpressed in pancreatic carcinoma cells and enhances tumor cell proliferation through transcriptional activation of the c-myc oncogene.

Methods: NFAT2, calcineurin and c-myc expression was assessed using real time PCR and Western blot analysis. NFAT2 activity was monitored by reporter gene assays, DNA binding studies and subcellular localization analysis. Endogenous NFAT2 activity was enhanced by stimulation with ionomycin or inhibited by cyclosporin A (CsA) treatment or siRNA-mediated knock-down of endogenous NFAT2. Effects of altered NFAT2 signaling were monitored by proliferation assays and FACS analysis.

Results: NFAT2 is ectopically expressed and activated in pancreatic cancer cells. CsA treatment led to inhibition of NFAT2 activity, indicating that Ca^{2+}/calcineurin signaling is required for the oncogenic activation of NFAT2. Activated NFAT2 directly binds to a specific element within the proximal c-myc promoter and up-regulates transcription of the c-myc oncogene. c-myc transcription and cell proliferation is significantly attenuated by inhibition of Ca^{2+}/calcineurin signaling or knock-down of NFAT2 expression. Overexpression of c-myc in NFAT2 knock-down cells fully restores the hyperproliferative phenotype.

Conclusions: Ectopic NFAT2 expression in combination with activation of the Ca^{2+}/calcineurin signaling pathway in pancreatic cancer cells results in a strong pro-proliferative effect in these cells. This effect is primarily mediated through the upregulation of the c-myc oncogene, ultimately resulting in accelerated G1/S phase transition and increased cell proliferation. Our results thus define a novel mechanism of oncogenic c-myc activation in pancreatic cancer cells.

9

PAP/Reg Inhibits Inflammation Through STAT3 Activation and IkappaB Upregulation in Pancreatic Epithelial Cells

E. Folch-Puy[1], S. Granell[1], J.-C. Dagorn[2], J.L. Iovanna[2], D. Closa[1]

[1]Dept. of Experimental Pathology, IIBB-CSIC, Barcelona, Spain; [2]Dept. Stress Cellulaire, INSERM U.624, Marseille, France

Introduction: PAP/Reg protein has been recently described as an endogenous mechanism involved in the regulation of inflammation. In the present study we show, for the first time, some of the molecular mechanisms involved in the intracellular signalling pathways activated by PAP/Reg in a pancreatic acinar cell line. Knowing that PAP/Reg and IL-10 responses share several features, we looked whether both could reciprocally regulate their expressions and whether JaK/STAT and NFkappaB signaling pathways were involved in the suppression of inflammation mediated by PAP/Reg.

Methods: AR42J cells were seeded at subconfluent levels and treated with immunopurified rat PAP/Reg or with IL-10. Total RNA was obtained 15 min, 30 min, 1 h, 2 h and 4 h after treatment and the expression of PAP/Reg, IL-10, IkappaB and SOCS-3 were examined by RT-PCR. In addition, STAT3 activation was measured by inmunofluorescence in cells activated with PAP/Reg. Western Blot analysis was used to determine the effect of PAP/Reg on STAT3 protein activation, SOCS3 and IkappaB expression.

Results: We observed a strong induction of PAP/Reg gene in response to IL-10 and, in response to PAP itself. PAP/Reg treatment induced phosphorylation and nuclear translocation of STAT3 while inhibited NFkappaB signaling pathway by overexpressing IkappaB. Finally, PAP/Reg exerts its effect through induction of the Supressor Of Cytokine Signaling (SOCS)3.

Conclusion: These findings suggest that PAP/Reg inhibits the inflammatory response through, at least two mechanisms, one dependent on STAT3 activation, the other targeting NFkappaB. Important functional similarities with the anti-inflammatory cytokine IL-10 suggests that PAP/Reg could be an IL-10 counterpart in epithelial cells.

10

Characterisation of H^+ and HCO_3^- Transporters in CFPAC-1 Human Pancreatic Duct Cells

Z. Rakonczay Jr.[1,2], A. Fearn[1], P. Hegyi[2,1], M.A. Gray[1], B.E. Argent[1]

[1]Institute for Cell and Molecular Biosciences, University of Newcastle upon Tyne, UK; [2]First Department of Medicine, University of Szeged, Hungary

Introduction: Pancreatic duct cells secrete an alkaline, HCO_3^- rich fluid, and this process is markedly reduced in cystic fibrosis (CF). Investigations of the H^+ and HCO_3^- transporters involved in ductal HCO_3^- secretion have been performed mainly on animal tissue. The aim

Table of Abstract 11

Follow up time (d)	Inflammation		Acinar cell vacuolization material		Acinar necrosis	
	Stent	Steel	Stent	Steel	Stent	Steel
0	0 [0–0]		0 [0–0]		0 [0–0]	
1	2 [1–3]	2 [1–2]	0 [0–0]	0 [0–0]	1 [1–1]	1 [0–1]
3	3 [2–3]	2 [1–3]	0 [0–0]	0 [0–0]	1 [1–4]	1 [0–4]
7	0.5 [0–2]	2 [1–3]	0 [0–0]	0 [0–0]	0 [0–0]	1 [0–3]*
21	0 [0–2]	0 [0–0]	0 [0–0]	0 [0–0]	0 [0–0]	0 [0–1]

Histological parameters scored from 0 to 4. Numbers in the table represent median [range].
*Radiopaque stent group vs. steel group: p = 0.028.

of this study was to characterize H^+ and HCO_3^- transporters in polarised CFPAC-1 human pancreatic duct cells (derived from a cystic fibrosis patient).

Methods: CFPAC-1 cells were seeded at high density onto permeable supports and grown to confluence. The cells were loaded with the pH sensitive fluorescent dye BCECF, and mounted into a perfusion chamber, which allowed the simultaneous perfusion of different solutions to the basolateral and apical membranes. Transmembrane base flux was calculated from changes in intracellular pH and the buffering capacity of the cells.

Results: The apical membrane of the cells is freely permeable to CO_2, but does not allow HCO_3^- influx from the lumen. In contrast, the basolateral membrane has transporters that allow rapid HCO_3^- entry into the cells. Our data show the functional presence of Na^+/H^+ exchangers on both the apical and basolateral membranes, and Cl^-/HCO_3^- exchanger and Na^+/HCO_3^- co-transporter activities on the basolateral membrane. 300 μM amiloride completely blocked Na^+/H^+ exchangers on both membranes of the cells. Basolateral HCO_3^- uptake was sensitive to variations of extracellular K^+ concentration and blocked by the anion transport inhibitor H_2-DIDS. Forskolin did not increase Cl^-/HCO_3^- exchange activities on the apical and basolateral membranes. The application of the membrane permeable carbonic anhydrase inhibitor, acetazolamide, partially decreased the rate of apical and basolateral acid flux and base flux, respectively.

Conclusions: These data suggest that polarised CFPAC-1 human pancreatic duct cells will be a useful model for studying HCO_3^- secretion in CF.

Funded by a Wellcome Trust Travelling Fellowship to Z.R. (069470), and a Wellcome Trust IRDA to P.H. (022618).

11

Bioabsorbable Stent Material (poly-L,D-Lactide-$BaSO_4$) is Biocompatible for Use in Pancreatic Applications – An Experimental Study

T. Lämsä[1], H. Jin[1], J. Mikkonen[2], J. Laukkarinen[1], J. Sand[1], I. Nordback[1]

[1]Department of Gastroenterology and Alimentary Tract Surgery, Tampere University Hospital, and [2]Institute of Biomaterials, Tampere University of Technology, Tampere Finland

Introduction: During the recent years we have been developing bioabsorbable biliary stents with very promising results. In developing pancreatic stents before long-term experiments, the acute toxicity of bioabsorbable, radiopaque polylactide (PLA-96-barium sulphate, $BaSO_4$) stent, to the pancreas was investigated in the present study.

Methods: Pancreas was exposed in 65 Sprague-Dawley rats either to radiopaque stent material (PLA-96 with 25% (w/w) of $BaSO_4$), radiolucent stent material (PLA-96) or steel by inserting a 5 mm long, 0.3 mm diameter fibre/stick of material into the pancreas in laparotomy under general anesthesia. Pancreatic tissue specimens and blood samples were taken after 1, 3, 7 and 21 days for histological determination and amylase activity measurement, respectively. Samples were also taken from 5 control rats without exposing to any materials.

Results: Control animals had normal serum amylase activity and had no histological changes in the pancreas. Radiopaque stent material (PLA-96-$BaSO_4$) induced an increase in the serum amylase activity (5845 u/l ± 1135 SE) at day 1, similar to the rats exposed to steel (4946 u/l ± 667 SE) and radiolucent stent material (PLA-96) (7684 u/l ± 739 SE). There was slightly more acinar cell necrosis on day 7 in the steel group than in the radiopaque stent (PLA-96-$BaSO_4$) group (Table).

Conclusions: Radiopaque stent material (PLA-96-$BaSO_4$) was not more toxic than the reference steel material in the rat pancreas during the 21-day observation period and is thus applicable for further in vivo experiments when developing pancreatic bioabsorbable stents.

12

Intragastric Ethanol Reduces Pancreatic Vascular Perfusion via an Endothelin-Mediated Mechanism

J.A. London[1], *C.M. Woods*[1], *C.J. Carati*[2], *J. Toouli*[1], *G.T.P. Saccone*[1]

[1]Department of General and Digestive Surgery, and [2]Department of Anatomy and Histology, Flinders Medical Centre, Flinders University, Australia

Introduction: Reduced pancreatic vascular perfusion (PVP) contributes to the development of necrosis in acute pancreatitis. Acute ethanol consumption can result in acute pancreatitis, however its effects on PVP have not been well characterized. The ethanol-induced change in PVP may involve endothelins. We have shown that intravenous ethanol does not change PVP.

Aim: To investigate the effects of intragastric (IG) ethanol on PVP in vivo and a possible role for endothelins.

Methods: Possums were anaesthetised (sodium thiopentone). Ethanol or water was instilled as an intragastric bolus (2 g/kg in water; 35% solution). In separate experiments the endothelin antagonist tezosentan (1 ml/kg/min at 3 ml/hr; Actelion Ltd) was administered as an intravenous infusion commencing 1 hour before the IG ethanol/water and continued for the duration of the experiment. Blood ethanol, blood pressure (BP) and PVP (Laser Doppler fluxmetry) in the head, body and tail of the pancreas were monitored over 4 hours.

Results: IG ethanol increased blood ethanol levels peaking at 275 ± 45 mg/100 mL. IG ethanol decreased PVP in the head, body and tail after 1hour to 61 ± 7, 58 ± 5 and 47 ± 9% of baseline respectively ($p < 0.05$). Generally PVP began to recover approximately 2.5 hours post-ethanol administration. There was no significant effect on BP. IG water did not alter BP or PVP. Treatment with tezosentan prevented the fall in PVP induced by ethanol.

Conclusion: These data suggests that IG ethanol reduces PVP, which could facilitate pancreatic damage. The tezosentan data suggests that the ethanol-induced PVP response is mediated by endothelins.

Supported by the NH&MRC of Australia (229901) and the FMC Foundation.

13

N-Terminal Processing of α1-Antitrypsin by Human Mesotrypsin

E. Szepessy, M. Sahin-Tóth

Department of Molecular and Cell Biology, Boston University Goldman School of Dental Medicine, Boston, MA, USA

Introduction: Human mesotrypsin does not form tight inhibitory complexes with natural polypeptide inhibitors and generally digests polypeptide substrates poorly. This unusual property is caused by Arg198, which interferes with substrate and inhibitor binding. Recently, we have shown that mesotrypsin rapidly cleaves the reactive-site peptide bond of the Kunitz-type soybean trypsin inhibitor and degrades the Kazal-type pancreatic secretory trypsin inhibitor. These observations established a physiological role for mesotrypsin in digestive degradation of dietary trypsin inhibitors and raised the possibility that it has a pathological role in the development of human pancreatitis. To extend these studies, we have characterized the interaction of mesotrypsin with the serum protease inhibitor α1-antitrypsin (α1AT), the prototype of the 'suicide-mechanism' serpin inhibitors.

Methods: Recombinant human α1AT and human trypsinogens were expressed in *Escherichia coli* and affinity purified. Native human α1AT was purchased from Sigma. Inhibitory activity and proteolytic cleavage of α1AT was followed by spectrophotometric trypsin assays, gel electrophoresis, Western blotting and N-terminal sequencing.

Results: Mesotrypsin did not form a covalent complex with α1AT, while anionic and cationic trypsins were readily complexed and inhibited. No competitive inhibition of mesotrypsin was observed with α1AT up to 20 μM concentration and mesotrypsin did not cleave the reactive-site peptide bond of α1AT. Unexpectedly, however, mesotrypsin rapidly proteolyzed the Lys10-Thr11 peptide bond of α1AT, which resulted in the release of the N-terminal decapeptide. The N-terminally processed α1AT retained its inhibitory activity toward cationic and anionic trypsins or neutrophil elastase.

Conclusions: The interaction between human mesotrypsin and α1AT follows a different paradigm than the previously described interactions with canonical trypsin inhibitors. Mesotrypsin does not recognize the Met358 reactive-site of α1AT, and thus exhibits essentially complete resistance to its inhibitory action. In turn, this allows specific and rapid N-terminal processing of α1AT, which formally categorizes α1AT as a novel natural substrate for mesotrypsin.

14

TIEG2 Plays a Key Role in the Cytostatic Program of TGFβ that is Selectively Lost in Pancreatic Cancer

A. Buck, J. Motzer, M. Buchholz, G. Adler, T.M. Gress, V. Ellenrieder

Department of Internal Medicine I, University of Ulm, Germany

Introduction: Smad3-mediated transcriptional repression of the c-myc oncogene is the initial key event in TGFβ-induced growth inhibition and is selectively lost in pancreatic cancer cells with activating K-Ras mutations. Here we examined the role of TIEG2 (KLF11) – a TGFβ-inducible transcriptional repressor- in this important function of TGFβ and studied how oncogenic Ras-signaling affects this interaction in pancreatic cancer cells refractory to TGFβ growth inhibition.

Methods: siRNA-technology was used to knock down endogenous TIEG2 expression. Promoter reporter studies, chromatin-immunoprecipitations, DNA-pulldown-assays and EMSA were conducted to study the role of TIEG2 in TGFβ-induced c-myc repression and growth inhibition. Co-immunopreciptiation studies were carried out to examine Smad3-TIEG2 complex formation and site-directed mutagenesis was used to identify Smad3-TIEG2 DNA binding sites within the c-myc promoter. Pharmacological inhibition of endogenous Erk-MAPK activation was performed in pancreatic cancer cells to elucidate the influence of oncogenic Ras-Mek-Erk signaling on TIEG2-Smad3 mediated c-myc repression.

Results: Depletion of endogenous TIEG2 expression causes loss of TGFβ-induced c-myc repression and renders epithelial cells resistant to TGFβ-induced growth inhibition. Mechanistically, TIEG2 interacts with TGFβ-activated Smad3 and cooperatively binds to and represses transcription from the recently identified TGFβ-inhibitory element (TIE) of the c-myc promoter. This novel mechanism in TGFβ growth inhibition is inhibited in pancreatic cancer cells in which oncogenic activation of the Ras-ERK signalling cascade leads to disruption of Smad3-TIEG2 complex formation on the c-myc promoter.

Conclusions: Our study reveals a novel mechanism in TGFβ growth inhibition which is defined by Smad3-TIEG2 mediated c-myc repression and is antagonized in pancreatic cancer cells through crosstalk with oncogenic Ras signalling.

15

Matrigel plus N-Acetylcysteine Deactivate Human Pancreatic Stellate Cells

R. Jesnowski[1,2], *D. Fürst*[1], *J. Ringel*[1], *J. Kleeff*[3], *A. Kolb*[3], *M. Löhr*[1,2]

[1]Department of Medicine II, Mannheim Medical Faculty, University of Heidelberg, Germany, [2]CCU Molecular Gastroenterology (E180), DKFZ, Heidelberg, Germany, [3]Department of Surgery, University of Heidelberg, Germany

Background/Aims: Tissue fibrosis is one of the characteristics of chronic pancreatitis and pancreatic adenocarcinoma. Activated pancreatic stellate cells (PSC) play a central role in this process. In the last years several factors resulting in activation of PSC have been identified, however, up to now no efficient therapy for the treatment of pancreatic fibrosis has been developed.

Methods: Primary activated pancreatic stellate cells were isolated by the outgrowth method. The effects of cultivation on basement membrane components or N-acetylcysteine (NAC) treatment on gene or protein expression and proliferation of primary activated human PSC and immortalized human PSC were analyzed. Methods used included RT-PCR and real-time RT-PCR, Western Blot and WST-1 assay. Fat storing of the cells was visualized by Oil Red staining and vitamin A autofluorescence.

Results: Incubation of immortalized and primary human activated PSC on Matrigel plus NAC treatment resulted in a deactivated phenotype as evidenced by a decrease of αSMA, CTGF and Col I expression and by a decreased proliferation of the cells. Moreover this treatment restored the ability of the cells to store vitamin A in cytoplasmic vesicles.

Conclusion: We were able to demonstrate that besides soluble factors, the matrix surrounding pancreatic stellate cells plays a pivotal role in the maintenance of the activation process of PSC. Cultivation of activated PSC on a reconstituted basement membrane plus treatment with NAC was able to deactivate the cells, thus pointing to the possibility of an antifibrosis therapy in chronic pancreatitis.

16

Cloning and Characterization of Genes Differentially Expressed in Human Pancreatic Carcinoma

Y. Chen[1,2], *R. Jesnowski*[1,2], *M. Löhr*[1,2]

[1]Section of Molecular Gastroenterology, Department of Medicine II, Faculty for Clinical Medicine Mannheim, University of Heidelberg, Germany, [2]Molecular Gastroenterology of German Cancer Research Center (DKFZ), Heidelberg, Germany

Introduction: Identification of 'novel' genes involved in pancreatic tumor progression is essential as a basis for the development of new treatment or diagnostic modalities. This study was about the cloning and characterization of full-length clones of several undefined partial cDNAs which were obtained by DDRT-PCR on RNA from patients with pancreatic cancer, chronic pancreatitis and normal pancreas from a former study of our group.

Methods: RACE (Rapid Amplification cDNA Ends) was performed for gene cloning. PANC-1 pancreatic cancer cells were stably transfected by the antisense constructs of genes upregulated in pancreatic carcinoma (ankyrin-B and SSR3). Down-regulation of the respective genes was comfirmed by RT-PCR, real time RT-PCR and Western Blot. Cell proliferation was determined by WST-1 and tumorigenic potential by soft agar assay. Cell migration and invasion capability was checked by Matrigel Basement Membrane coated transwells.

Results: By RACE-PCR, we obtained the full-length cDNAs of the undefined clones. Transfection of antisense constructs of the two above-mentioned genes decreased their expression on RNA level, ankyrin B down-regulation was also seen on protein level. The antisense clones exhibited a reduction of growth rate of about 30% and an average colony forming efficacy of 60% for ankyrin-B and 76% for SSR3 antisense clones compared to the parental cells. Transfected Ank-B and SSR3 cells were attenuated the ability of migration and invasion.

Conclusion: Our findings document that ankyrin-B and SSR3 are overexpressed in pancreatic cancer and that the suppression of these genes expression attenuates the growth potential of pancreatic cancer cells and some tumor characteristics. The identification of several pancreatic cancer related 'novel' genes which have never been studied in pancreatic carcinoma before may be contribute to the gene therapy of pancreatic disease.

17

The Eph/Ephrin Signaling System in the Mouse Pancreas

A. Merlos-Suárez[1,2], *E. Batlle*[3], *N. Rafel*[1,2], *R. Bort*[1,2], *F.X. Real*[1,2]

[1]D. Ciències Experimentals i de la Salut, Universitat Pompeu Fabra, [2]Institut Municipal d'Investigació Mèdica, [3]Parc Científic de Barcelona-ICREA, Barcelona, Spain

Introduction: The cell types coexisting in the pancreas are organized in functionally different compartments. It is not known how the boundaries of these compartments are established during development and further maintained in adulthood. The Eph kinase receptor family (Ephs) and their ligands, the ephrins (Efn), participate in patterning and morphogenetic processes in several tissues. We investigated the expression of Ephs and ephrins in the mouse pancreas and their possible role in the formation and maintenance of boundaries in this organ.

Methods: Immunohistochemistry, in situ hybridization, and quantitative RT-PCR were performed on embryonic and adult mouse pancreata to study the expression patterns of Ephs and ephrins.

Results: During embryonic pancreas development the expression of Ephs and ephrins was found to be dynamically regulated; the levels of EphA1, EphA2 and EphA8 mRNAs increased, while EphA4, EfnA4, EfnA5 and EfnB3 were downregulated as development progressed. In the adult, Ephs and ephrins displayed distinct patterns of expression in the exocrine and endocrine pancreas; receptors A5 and A7 were found to be highly expressed in the acinar cells, while none of the receptors or ligands studied showed a ductal cell-restricted pattern. These findings are consistent with a role of Ephs and ephrins in boundary formation and maintenance in the pancreas.

Conclusions: Ephs and ephrins display distinct expression patterns in pancreatic cells. As in other epithelia, this signaling system may be required for the correct cellular organization in the pancreas. Ephrin knock-out mice are currently being investigated to definitely establish this hypothesis.

18

Basolateral pNBC1 and NHE1 Regulate Intracellular pH and Transepithelial Bicarbonate Secretion in Capan-1 Cells

A. Szűcs[1], I. Demeter[1], G. Ovári[1], R.M. Case[2], M.C. Steward[2], G. Varga[1]

[1]Molecular Oral Biology Research Group, Hungarian Academy of Sciences and Semmelweis University, Budapest, Hungary; [2]Faculty of Life Sciences, University of Manchester, UK

Aim: The present study sought to identify the transporters that maintain intracellular pH (pH_i) during pancreatic transepithelial bicarbonate secretion.

Methods: The expression of potential key transporters and receptors was compared in normal human pancreas and in cultured Capan-1 human pancreatic ductal cells by RT-PCR. Polarised monolayers of Capan-1 cells were grown on Transwell-COL PTFE membranes. To estimate transmembrane and transcellular bicarbonate movements, pH_i was monitored by microfluorometry using BCECF, a pH-sensitive fluoroprobe. Bicarbonate secretion was estimated from the initial rate of decrease in intracellular pH (pH_i) following inhibition of basolateral bicarbonate uptake by EIPA (to block basolateral Na^+-H^+ exchange) and H_2DIDS (to inhibit Na^+-HCO_3^- cotransport).

Results: By RT-PCR we found that pNBC1, NHE1, AE2, AE3, SLC26A6 transporters, CFTR channel and secretin, VPAC1, P2Y1,2,4,6 receptors were expressed both in normal human pancreas and in Capan-1 cells. In functional studies the initial rate of recovery of pH_i following the NH_4CI pulse was almost completely inhibited by basolateral but not by apical application of the EIPA and H_2DIDS. Simultaneous administration of basolateral EIPA and H_2DIDS led to an immediate, significant decrease in pH_i (0.06667 ± 0.00281 pH/min) compared to untreated control (0.00001 ± 0,00005 pH/min). The initial decrease in pH_i was accelerated by apical ATP (0.10403 ± 0.00448 pH/min) or UTP and inhibited by basolateral ATP (0.00088 ± 0.00009 pH/min) or UTP administration. Forskolin, secretin and VIP also stimulated vectorial bicarbonate secretion.

Conclusions: NBC and NHE are present in both normal human pancreas and in Capan-l cells. In Capan-1 cells NBC and NHE, localised exclusively at the basolateral membrane, are the key transporters involved in the maintenance of pH_i both during cellular acidification and during transcellular bicarbonate secretion. Extracellular purinergic activation induces differential effects, stimulation at the apical side, and inhibition on the basolateral side.

19

Matrigel Induces Ductal-Acinar Transdifferentiation in HSG Epithelial Cell Line

V. Szlávik, K. Nagy, G. Varga

Molecular Oral Biology Research Group, Hungarian Academy of Sciences and Semmelweis University, Budapest, Hungary

Introduction: Acinar cells of exocrine glands are responsible for secretion of sufficient amount of electrolytes, water and digestive enzymes. Ductal cells, regarded to be ontogenetically preceding cell types, form structural elements of the canal system of epithelial glands and modify primary secretion. The present study was designed to examine in vitro acinar transdifferentiation of human ductal derived HSG cells, and the characterization of this process.

Methods: HSG cells were cultivated in DMEM supplemented 10% FCS under standard conditions and in Matrigel matrix. Plated cells were fixed for microscopical studies to study morphological changes. The gene expression pattern of normal and differentiated HSG cells was compared by RT-PCR. DNA synthesis during the transdifferentiation process was followed by ^{3}H-thymidine incorporation.

Results: Under standard culture conditions, grown on plastic surface, HSG cells of ductal origin formed epitheloid fields and proliferated continually. Matrigel matrix containing extracellular matrix components led HSG cells to form acinar structures, and to develop dense luminar microvilli system and Golgi complex. DNA synthesis of HSG cells grown in Matrigel was 18 ± 11% of that of control cells (100 ± 8%) cultured on plastic surface ($p < 0.05$) after 24 h in culture, clearly suggesting an inhibition of proliferative activity during differentiation. Parallel to these changes, expression of amylase, syndecan and electrolyte transporters pancreatic Na^+/HCO_3^- cotransporter 1 (pNBC1), Na^+-dependent chloride transporter (NKCC1) and Cl^-/HCO_3^- exchanger pendrin (SLC26A4) expression have also differentially changed in HSG cells.

Conclusions: The HSG cell line is a suitable in vitro model system to study cell biological mechanisms of ductal-acinar transdifferentiation of exocrine gland cells and to examine transporter molecules responsible for acinar and ductal functions.

20

Proteomic Identification of Two New Proteins Secreted by Pancreatic Cancer Cells: Versican and MAC25/Angiomodulin

A. Bonora[1], M. Della Peruta[2], P. Mauri[3], G. Maraia[1], A. Cavallini[1], A. Mafficini[2], C. Bassi[1], A. Scarpa[2], P. Pederzoli[1], C. Sorio[2]

[1]Department of Surgical Sciences and [2]Department of Pathology, University of Verona, Italy, [3]Institute of Biomedical Technologies (ITB-CNR), Milan, Italy

Introduction: The development of new approaches like Multidimensional Protein Identification Technology (MudPIT) made proteomics a more effective tool in detecting and analysing new markers which could be critical for better understand the biology of cancer and improve its detection in early and non invasive stage.

Methods: We focused our investigation on pancreatic cancer cell line SUIT-2, in order to firstly identify the proteins secreted and released by pancreatic cancer cells. We analyzed with MudPIT small amounts of serum-free supernatant, produced by cultured SUIT-2 cells. The analysis was broadened using RT-PCR in a series of pancreatic carcinoma cell lines and xenografts. Moreover, immunohistochemistry in both primary pancreatic cancers and in SUIT-2 cells embedded in Matrigel and implanted in nude mice was performed to confirm the production and release of the proteins in the extracellular matrix.

Results: Forty seven largely secreted proteins were identified. Out of these, Chondroitin sulphate proteoglycan 2 (CSPG2/Versican) and MAC25/Angiomodulin (MAC25/IGFBP-rP1/IGFBP7) had never been previously described as released by pancreatic cancer cells. Nine of 19 (47%) cell lines appeared positive for CSPG2 and seven (37%) for MAC25 mRNA. The 93% (14/15) of xenografts were positive for CSPG2 mRNAs, while 12 (80%) for MAC25. In both primary pancreatic cancers and in Matrigel-embedded SUIT-2 cells immunohistochemistry confirmed the in vivo production and release of the proteins in the extracellular matrix.

Conclusion: CSPG2/Versican and MAC25/Angiomodulin are secreted by pancreatic cancer cells, both in vitro and in vivo. Therefore, CSPG2 is not only a 'marker' of the stromal reaction typical of pancreatic cancer, but it appears to be actively synthesized by cancer cells and stored in the extracellular milieu, this suggesting a possible role in the mechanism of tumour-host defense. The role of MAC25 in pancreatic carcinoma is still unknown and requires further investigations.

21

Phorbol Esters and Regulatory Peptides Control DNA Synthesis by Activating Several Protein Kinase C Isoforms in Panc-1 Cancer Cells

G. Varga, B. Burghardt, V. Szlávik, G.Z. Rácz

Molecular Oral Biology Research Group, Department of Oral Biology, Hungarian Academy of Sciences and Semmelweis University, Budapest, Hungary

Background: Previously we have shown that ERK plays a key role in the growth regulatory effects of regulatory peptides and PKC activation in human pancreatic cancer cells. Now we studied the temporal pattern of the activation of different PKC isoforms in response to stimulation with regulatory peptides or phorbol ester treatment. We also investigated the effect of PKC activation on the ERK cascade and the DNA synthesis in Panc-1 cells.

Methods: Panc-1 cells transfected with CCK1 receptors (Panc-1C) were treated with 10 nM cholecystokinin (CCK), 50 nM neurotensin (NT) or 100 nM phorbol 12-myristate 13-acetate (PMA). DNA synthesis was studied by measuring tritiated thymidine incorporation. PKC isoforms were selectively inhibited with 20 nM Gö6983 (a, b, g, d) or 200 nM Ro-32-0432 (a, b, g, e), their translocation was detected by confocal microscopy and by subcellular fractionation followed by immunoblotting. ERK cascade activation was detected with phosphoERK immunoblotting. PKCe-Raf1 complexes were detected by immunoprecipitation and western blotting.

Results: PMA and CCK inhibits, whereas NT stimulates DNA synthesis. Inhibition is mediated by long term, while stimulation is mediated by transient ERK activation. These effects are prevented by Ro-32-0432 but not by Gö6983. Confocal microscopy and subcellular fractionation demonstrates that PMA causes cytosol to nuclear and cytosol to membrane translocation, whereas CCK and NT cause cytosol-membrane translocation of PKCa, -d and -e over a time course ranging from 2 to 30 minutes. ERK activation is inhibited by Ro-32-0432 but not by Gö6983. PKCe is detected in Raf1 immunoprecipitates.

Conclusion: Exposure of Panc-1C cells to the regulatory peptides CCK or NT or the phorbol ester PMA induces the translocation of PKCa, -d and -e and regulates DNA synthesis in a PKCe-dependent manner. ERK activation induced by PMA or by regulatory peptides depends on PKCe.

22

Functional Analysis of S100A6 (Calcyclin) in Pancreatic Cancer Patients

T. Nedjadi[1], *D. Vimalachandran*[1], *C.C.M. Thompson*[1], *J. Lüttges*[2], *W. Prime*[3], *F. Campbell*[4], *A. Dodson*[4], *T. Crnogorac-Jurcevic*[5], *N.R. Lemoine*[5], *W. Greenhalf*[1], *J.P. Neoptolemos*[1], *E. Costello*[1]

[1]Division of Surgery and Oncology, University of Liverpool, UK; [2]Department of Pathology, UKSH, Kiel, Germany; [3]Cancer Tissue Bank Research Centre, Department of Pathology, University of Liverpool, UK, [4]Department of Pathology, Royal Liverpool University Hospital, Liverpool, UK, [5]Cancer Research UK Clinical Centre, Queen Mary's School of Medicine at Barts & The London, John Vane Science Building, London, UK

Introduction: Recent studies, including our own, have reported elevated levels of the calcium binding protein, S100A6, in malignant cells in pancreatic ductal adenocarcinoma. The aim of the current study was to analyse the expression of S100A6 in benign, malignant and pre-malignant pancreatic ductal cells and to correlate this with clinical and pathological parameters. In addition, we aimed to determine whether S100A6 contributes to the motility of pancreatic cancer cells.

Methods: S100A6 expression was determined by immunohistochemical analysis in benign (n = 32), malignant (n = 60) and pre-malignant pancreatic ductal cells (96 pancreatic intraepithelial neoplasias (PanINs) from 46 patients) and levels of expression were correlated with clinical and pathological parameters. RNA interference was used to knockdown S100A6 expression in three pancreatic cancer cell lines and cell motility assessed.

Results: S100A6 staining was more intense in malignant than in benign cells (p = 0.0001). In malignant cells, staining was higher in the nucleus than the cytoplasm (p = 0.003). Univariate analysis revealed a significant decrease in survival time for patients with high levels of nuclear (p = 0.01), but not cytoplasmic (p = 0.20) S100A6. Analysis of PanIN lesions revealed a general absence of S100A6 staining in PanIN 1a lesions. Thereafter, there was a progressive increase in the proportion of positively stained PanINs with increasing PanIN grade. Knockdown of S100A6 was accompanied by a reduction in the motility of pancreatic cancer cells.

Conclusion: The data suggest that upregulation of S100A6 is an early event in pancreatic cancer development and that elevated levels of nuclear S100A6 may affect clinical outcome. It is possible that S00A6 contributes to the motility of pancreatic cancer cells.

23

The K7 Promoter as a Strategy to Target Transgenes to Pancreatic Ductal Cells in vitro and in vivo

F.X. Real[1,2], *J. Pujal*[1], *I. Abasolo*[1], *A. Rodolosse*[1,2], *A. Duch*[1,2], *F.J.D. Smith*[3], *W.H.I. McLean*[3]

[1]Unitat de Biologia Cellular i Molecular, Institut Municipal d'Investigació Mèdica; [2]Universitat Pompeu Fabra, Barcelona, Spain; [3]Ninewells Medical School, Dundee, UK

Introduction: Keratin 7 (K7) is a type II polypeptide expressed in selected cell types in a variety of simple epithelia, including the pancreas, biliary system, kidney, and bladder. K7 is absent from the epithelium lining the human gastrointestinal tract. Interestingly, K7 is expressed exclusively in ductal cells but not in other pancreatic cell types.

Methods: We have used deletion constructs of the *krt2–7* promoter in transient transfection reporter assays and have produced mutant reported plasmids to analyze the role of Sp1-like binding sites. Transgenic mice expressing LacZ under the control of the *krt2–7* promoter have been generated.

Results: All elements required for the maintenance of appropriate tissue specificity in vitro are present within the −234 bp sequence. This fragment confers a >50-fold higher activity in pancreatic ductal cells than in pancreatic acinar cells and 30-fold more specific reporter activity than the *krt1–19* promoter when comparing human pancreatic ductal cells with intestinal cells. The sequence of the promoters of mouse and human genes coding for K7 contained GC-rich sequences corresponding to putative Sp1, AP-2 binding sequences, among others. Mutant reporter plasmids showed that these sites are essential for the in vitro activity of the promoter. Particularly, occupancy of the Sp1-like sequences was confirmed by electrophoretic mobility shift assays though differential binding of nuclear proteins to these elements was found not to be responsible for the cell type-specificity. K7-LacZ transgenic mice displayed high levels of beta-galactosidase activity in normal pancreatic ducts.

Conclusion: These results provide the rationale to use the proximal region of the murine *krt2–7* promoter to target transgenes into pancreatic ductal cells in vivo, thus being of potential importance for the study of pancreatic biology and pathology in mouse models.

24

Impact of SMAD4 Reconstitution on Expression of Angiogenetic Factors and ECM Proteins in BxPC-3 Cells

A. Schrödel, M. Russcher, R. Jesnowski, M. Löhr

Clinical Cooperation Unit of Molecular Gastroenterology, DKFZ, Heidelberg, and II. Med. Klinik Mannheim, Germany

Introduction: Loss of SMAD4 in pancreatic adenocarcinoma is associated with the transition to an invasive and metastatic phenotype. SMAD proteins are involved in TGF-β signalling. TGF-β induces e.g. the synthesis of VEGF and extracellular matrix (ECM). The effect of

SMAD4 re-constitution on angiogenesis and ECM formation was tested in BxPC-3 cells.

Methods: We used BxPC-3 cells and immortal pancreatic stellate cells (PSC). SMAD4 re-constituted (SMAD4+) and SMAD4 deficient (SMAD4–) control cells were stimulated with TGFβ-1 in culture medium without FCS. RNA was isolated to perform RT-PCR.

Results: An increase in expression of anti-angiogenetic factor TSP-1 (Thrombospondin-1) and a decrease in VEGF expression was seen in SMAD4+ cells. SPARC, an anti-adhesive glycoprotein of the ECM, Fibronectin and CTGF (connective tissue growth factor) were induced by TGFβ-1 in SMAD4+ as well as in SMAD4– cells, and the level of induction was higher in the SMAD4+ cells. Expression of the ECM proteins laminin and collagen-I was higher in the SMAD4– cells but was independent of TGFβ-1 stimulation. The pancreatic stellate cells showed much more fibronectin and SPARC mRNA in contrast to the BxPC-3 cells.

Conclusion: We were able to confirm previous results on angiogenesis by SMAD4 positive cells in a different cell type. Therefore we suggest that this might be a general phenomenon. Biological functions of SPARC appear to be variable among different cancer types. We detected an upregulation of SPARC in the BxPC-3 SMAD4+ cells while it was postulated that SPARC expression in SW480 cells was suppressed by SMAD4. Furthermore it is generally accepted in the literature that CTGF stimulates the production of collagen, fibronectin and laminin. Here, CTGF was overexpressed in the SMAD4+ cells, but collagen-I was not. When the SMAD4+ were co-cultivated with pancreatic stellate cells, no increase of collagen-I production in either of the cells could be detected.

25

The Actin Capping Protein, CapG, is Overexpressed in Pancreatic Cancer and Modulates Motility in Pancreatic Cancer Cell Lines

C.C.M. Thompson[1], F.J. Ashcroft[1], S. Patel[1], G. Saraga[1], D. Vimalachandran[1], F. Campbell[2], N.R. Lemoine[3], J.P. Neoptolemos[1], E. Costello[1]

[1]Division of Surgery and Oncology, University of Liverpool, UK, [2]Department of Pathology, University of Liverpool, [3]Cancer Research UK Molecular Oncology Unit, Barts and the London School of Medicine and Dentistry, London, UK

Introduction: Extensive local invasion and metastatic spread are characteristics of pancreatic ductal adenocarcinoma, although little is known about the mechanisms that operate in such processes. Here, we describe the overexpression of a cell motility-associated actin capping protein, CapG, in malignant pancreatic ductal cells and its effect on cell motility in pancreatic cancer cell lines in vitro.

Methods: CapG was identified by mass spectrometry from spots excised from two-dimensional (2-D) electrophoresis gels and confirmed by 2-D immunoblotting. Expression in benign ($n = 44$) and malignant ($n = 69$) pancreatic tissue sections was examined by immunohistochemistry (IHC) on a pancreas cancer tissue microarray. CapG levels in three pancreatic cancer cell lines, Suit-2, MiaPaCa-2 and Panc-1, were reduced using RNA interference. Cell motility in these lines was assessed by measuring cell translocation across 8 micrometre porous membranes.

Results: CapG appeared as several isoforms on 2-D gels and immunoblots, possibly representing post-translationally modified forms of the protein. IHC analysis showed significantly higher staining intensity in both nuclear ($p < 0.0001$, Mann-Whitney U-test) and cytoplasmic ($p < 0.0001$) compartments of malignant, compared to benign, ductal cells. A significant ($p = 0.03$) association was identified between nuclear, but not cytoplasmic, CapG and tumour size. Reducing CapG levels resulted in a significant reduction in cell motility in MiaPaCa-2 and Suit-2 cells. No significant reduction was observed in Panc-1 experiments.

Discussion: The identification of proteins involved in the phenotype of pancreatic cancer cells will lead to an improved understanding of the mechanistic basis of cancer cell invasion. Our evidence that CapG is overexpressed in pancreatic cancer and that it can modulate cell motility in vitro suggests that it may function as part of the invasive phenotype and perhaps promote the dissemination of pancreatic cancer cells.

This work is supported by Cancer Research UK and the North West Cancer Research Fund.

26

Dose-Dependent Effects of LPS and TNF-α on Intravascular, Transendothelial and Extravascular Leukocyte Locomotion

E. Ryschich, P. Lizdenis, V. Kerkadze, H.-P. Knaebel, M.W. Büchler, J. Schmidt

Dept. of Surgery, University of Heidelberg, Germany

Introduction: The ability for active movement is an important feature of leukocytes. Most migration assays do not allow the continuous visualisation of leukocyte locomotion in vivo. Here, we utilized a modified technique which combines intravital microscopy and time-elapsed video documentation to investigate leukocyte movement and the effect of pro-inflammatory stimuli in vivo.

Methods: Intravital microscopy of mesenterial tissue was performed in 30 male Lewis-rats using digital imaging and time-elapsed video compression. The number of rolling and crawling leukocytes, leukocyte transmigration, leukocyte velocity and the number of migrating leukocytes were measured over 60 min. The local effect of LPS and TNF-α on intra- and extravascular leukocyte movement was investigated.

Results: Adherent leukocytes showed an active intraluminal crawling along the endothelial lining, whereas only single leukocytes migrated through the endothelium without stimulation. Baseline measurement showed a mean velocity of the extravascular leukocytes of 9.9 ± 1.1 μm/min and a mean percentage of migrating cells of $83.7 \pm 3.3\%$. Concentration of LPS up to 20 μg/ml and concentration of TNF-α up to 50 ng/ml significantly activated the leukocyte locomotion in a dose-dependent manner, whereas higher concentrations significantly decreased the migratory activity of extravascular leukocytes.

Conclusions: Intravascular leukocyte crawling may precede, but does not always lead to transmigration. Low doses of LPS and TNF-α activated intraluminal, transendothelial and extravascular leukocyte migration. However, high concentrations of LPS and TNF-α inhibit leukocyte locomotion which can represent a relevant immunosuppressive factor in sepsis and infections.

27

Vitamin E Sensitizes Pancreatic Stellate (PSCs) Cells to Tumor Necrosis Factor (TNF)-α Induced Death through a Nuclear Factor (NF)-κB-Independent Mechanism

M. Rickmann, E. Vaquero, X. Molero, J.R. Malagelada

Digestive System Research Unit, Hospital Universitari Vall d'Hebron, Barcelona, Spain

Introduction: A hallmark of chronic pancreatitis is the pseudotumoral expansion of PSCs. Induction of PSC apoptosis may halt the progression of the disease. NF-κB is a redox-sensitive transcription factor critical in the anti-apoptotic pathway initiated by TNF-α.

Aims: To investigate the effects of vitamin E on intracellular ROS, apoptosis and NF-κB in PSCs exposed to TNF-α.

Methods: Rat PSCs were treated with vitamin E (α-tocopherol, 200 μM) for 72 h with or without TNF-α (20 ng/ml). Intracellular ROS were measured by flow cytometry using DCFH-DA/PI (propidium iodide); apoptosis was assessed by caspase-3 activity and DNA fragmentation; NF-κB was analyzed by ELISA quantification of p50 and p65 in nuclear extracts.

Results: PSCs had a basal level of endogenous ROS that was efficiently reduced by vitamin E after 48 h (40% of basal) and 72 h (30% of basal). To exclude the effects of cell toxicity on ROS analysis, necrotic cells (PI+) were eliminated from cytometric evaluation. TNF-α induced a time-dependent increase of ROS that reached 4-fold above basal levels at 72 h and that was abrogated with vitamin E. TNF-α and vitamin E by themselves did not induce apoptosis. However, in cells pretreated with vitamin E for 48 h TNF-α caused a 3-fold increase in DNA fragmentation, suggesting that ROS may protect PSCs from apoptosis. TNF-α caused a rapid and sustained NF-κB activation that could not be prevented with vitamin E. In order to suppress TNF-α induced NF-κB activation, MG-132 (NF-κB inhibitor) or cycloheximide (protein synthesis inhibitor) were added to vitamin E. This combination further enhanced the proapoptotic action of TNF-α.

Conclusions: Vitamin E renders PSCs susceptible to TNF-α induced apoptosis. This action cannot be ascribed to inhibition of the NF-κB pathway. Combined strategies aiming to reduce endogenous ROS levels and NF-κB activation might be beneficial to eliminate PSCs in chronic pancreatitis.

28

Membrane-Bound NAD(P)H Oxidase Repressess Cytotoxic Effects of Tumor Necrosis Factor (TNF)-α in Pancreatic Stellate Cells (PSCs)

E. Vaquero, M. Rickmann, X. Molero, J.R. Malagelada

Digestive System Research Unit, Hospital Universitari Vall d'Hebron, Barcelona, Spain

Introduction: In many non-phagocytic cells NADP(H) oxidase generates radical oxygen species (ROS) as critical survival signaling intermediates. PSCs, the main cell type responsible for pancreatic fibrosis, are activated upon oxidative conditions. TNF-α is a redox-responsive molecule that induces pro-survival responses in PSCs.

Aim: To study if membrane-associated NADP(H) oxidase is activated by TNF-α and its role in precluding PSC death.

Methods: PSCs isolated from rat pancreas were preincubated for 30 min with the NAD(P)H oxidase inhibitor dyphenilene iodonium (DPI) and then stimulated with TNF-α for defined periods of time (1 h, 3 h, 6 h, 24 h). NADP(H) oxidase activity was measured on membrane fractions by lucigenin chemiluminescence. Cell death was assessed by DNA fragmentation; caspase-8 and -3 activities; and flow cytometric assays using fluorescein diacetate (FDA) and propidium iodide (PI) for apoptotic and necrotic death and DiOC6(3)/PI for mitochondrial membrane potential.

Results: TNF-α significantly stimulated NADP(H) oxidase activity for the entire observation period, and this effect was abolished by DPI. TNF-α by itself did not elicit cell death. On the contrary, DPI stimulated PSC death, as indicated by a significant increase in DNA fragmentation, caspase activation, FDA–/PI– cells (apoptotic cells), FDA–/PI+ cells (late apoptotic/primary necrotic cells), and reduction of mitochondrial membrane potential. Interestingly, DPI greatly sensitize PSCs to TNF-α induced death, suggesting that ROS derived from NAD(P)H oxidase are hampering the pro-apoptotic potential of TNF-α. Inhibition of the upstream caspase-8 by IETD-fmk totally blocked DPI-sensitization of TNF-α induced apoptosis. Thus, the sensitizing effect of DPI is mediated by the extrinsic, and not the mitochondrial, death pathway and involves processing of caspase-8 and -3.

Conclusions: TNF-α stimulates ROS production in PSCs by an NAD(P)H oxidase-dependent mechanism. This pro-oxidative effect silences the cytotoxic actions of TNF-α. NADP(H) oxidase can be an useful therapeutic target in the treatment of pancreatic fibrosis by facilitating PSC elimination.

29

CD38 Antigen, a Key Player in NAADP Production and CCK Responses in Pancreatic Exocrine Cells

N. Cheviron[1], A. Menteyne[1], F.E. Lund[2], M.J. Moutin[3], J.M. Cancela[1]

[1]CNRS, Neurobiologie Cellulaire et Moléculaire, Gif-sur-Yvette, France; [2]Trudeau Institute, NY, USA; [3]Laboratoire des canaux ioniques et signalisation EMI99-31, INSERM, DRDC-CEA, Grenoble, France

Introduction: In pancreatic exocrine cells, the hormone cholecystokinin (CCK) and acetylcholine (ACh) induces specific Ca^{2+} signals. Receptors for the second messengers inositol-trisphosphate (IP_3) and cyclic ADPribose (cADPR) are known to be involved in CCK and ACh induced calcium signalling. In addition, nicotinic acid adenine dinucleotide phosphate (NAADP) receptor is specifically involved in CCK-evoked Ca^{2+} signals. It is known that ACh uses the ADP-ribosylcyclase, CD38, for cADPR synthesis whereas CCK uses another ADPribosyl cyclase for cADPR production. Moreover, it has been proposed that the CD38 is able to synthesize NAADP.

Methods: Our work has focussed on determining whether CD38 is responsible for synthesizing NAADP in pancreatic exocrine cells. This enzyme uses NADP as a substrate and catalyses the exchange of nicotinamide group with nicotinic acid, producing NAADP. This reaction can be monitored using HPLC, to quantify NAADP synthesis and measure enzyme specific activity. Assays performed with pancreatic extracts from control mice revealed NAADP production (12 nmol NAADP/mg protein/min), however, in contrast, NAADP synthesis could not be detected in extracts prepared from CD38-knock out mice.

Results: To elucidate the role of CD38 in hormone-induced intracellular calcium, signalling, we used conventional and confocal microscopy. Transgenic CD38−/− cells showed no responses to application of ACh 25 and 100 nM (n = 23/29; 22/24, respectively) and to application of 5 and 50 pM CCK (n = 28/33; 23/26, respectively). In contrast control cells displayed very frequent responses (n = 17/20, 12/16, 14/17, 13/15, respectively). In the rare cases of CD38−/− responsive cells, the responses recorded were with a much longer latency and with no Ca^{2+} oscillations. CD38−/− cells responded to application of high concentration of CCK (1 nM) suggesting that the IP_3 pathway remain functional (n = 5/5).

Conclusions: These results further support our hypothesis that CD38 is responsible for NAADP synthesis in vivo and that NAADP is an important second messenger in pancreatic exocrine cells.

30

Regulation of Exocrine Pancreas in Pigs with Normal and Retarded Growth

S. Rengman, B.W. Weström, S.G. Pierzynowski

Department of Cell and Organism Biology, Lund University, Sweden

Introduction: The relationship between exocrine pancreas function and growth has been neglected and seldom discussed. The aim of the studies was to show pancreas regulation via CCK_1 and CCK_2 receptors in pigs with normal and retarded growth.

Methods: The experiment was performed on six pigs, anaesthetised with ketamine, and surgically prepared for pancreatic juice collection and iv infusions. The pigs were born within a five-day period, and weighed between 14 and 42 kg at the time of the experiment. In order to maintain a steady secretion of pancreatic juice, 10 pmol/kg/h secretin was continuously infused intravenously during the experiment. After two 10 min control collection periods, CCK-33 was administered, first locally (13 pmol/kg) as a bolus to the duodenum/stomach arterial circulation, and than peripherally, to the jugular vein (130 pmol/kg). Pancreatic juice was collected in two 5 min and two 10 min periods after each treatment. All experiments were repeated after bilateral vagotomy.

Results: The exocrine pancreatic secretion (as protein and trypsin levels) showed a different pattern in the pigs with retarded growth in comparison to that of normally growing animals. Namely, the pigs with retarded growth did not respond to peripheral stimulation with CCK-33, which activates CCK_1 receptors (Evilevitch et al., Scand J Gastroenterol 2003;38:201–206). All pigs responded equally to the local infusion of CCK-33 in low-physiological doses, which mainly activates CCK_2 receptors (Evilevitch et al., Scand J Gastroenterol 2004;39:886–890). Vagotomy did not change the pattern of these responses.

Conclusions: The results suggested that a lack of response to the peripherally administered high-pharmacological dose of CCK-33 in the slow growing pigs might be related to a dysfunction of CCK_1 receptors.

31

Encapsulation of a Hamster Pancreatic Islet Cell Line in Sodium Cellulose Sulfate

V. Stadlbauer[1], P. Stiegler[2], S. Schaffellner[2], G. Halwachs[3], O. Hauser[4], F. Iberer[2], K.H. Tscheliessnigg[2], C. Lackner[5]

[1]Department of Internal Medicine, [2]Department of Surgery, [3]Department of Laboratory Medicine, Medical University of Graz, [4]Austrianova, Vienna; [5]Institute of Pathology, Medical University of Graz, Austria

Introduction: Diabetes mellitus will affect more than 150 million people worldwide in the near future. Late diabetic complications cannot be prevented by conventional insulin therapy due to recurrent peaks of elevated blood glucose levels. Therefore new therapeutic concepts of insulin replacement therapy such as pancreas transplantation are evolving. Due to shortage of human pancreas donor organs, transplantation of microencapsulated xenogeneic pancreas islets has attracted considerable attention. Microencapsulation using polyethylene-glycane or other polymers has been shown to sufficiently protect xenogeneic cells from host immune response but shortens life span of encapsulated cell after transplantation. Sodium cellulose sulfate (NaCS) is a novel polymer without unfavourable effect on cell survival. NaCS has not yet been tested for encapsulation of pancreatic beta-cells.

Methods: An insulin-producing, immortalized, hamster pancreatic beta-cell line (HIT-T15) was cultured in Ham-F12 and cells were encapsulated in NaCS in cooperation with Austrianova, Vienna. Cell growth and vitality was assessed with a MTT (3-[4,5-dimethylthiazol-2-yl]-2,5-diphenyltetrazolium bromide) based cell growth determination kit; the number of apoptotic cells was determined semiquantitatively by immunocytochemistry using antibodies against caspase 3 and 8; glucose dependent insulin secretion was assessed using ELISA in encapsulated and non-encapsulated HIT-T15 cells.

Results: Encapsulated and non-encapsulated cells showed comparable glucose dependent cell growth and apoptosis rates. Stimulation of HIT-T15 cells with glucose (20 mg/ml) resulted in a typically biphasic insulin secretion response with a first peak after 5 or 8 min and a second peak after 40 or 50 min (non-encapsulated and encapsulated cells, respectively).

Conclusions: Our results show that encapsulation of HIT-T15 cells in NaCS does not alter cell growth and vitality. Glucose stimulation resulted in a biphasic insulin secretion response which compares well to insulin responsiveness observed under physiological conditions in humans (non-encapsulated cells) or exogenous insulin therapy (encapsulated cells). Our results suggest that NaCS is well suited for microencapsulation of pancreatic beta-cells.

Experimental Acute and Chronic Pancreatitis

32

Hydrogen Sulfide Plays a Key Role in the Pathogenesis of Acute Pancreatitis and Associated Lung Injury

M. Bhatia, F.L. Wong, D. Fu, H.Y. Lau, S.M. Moochhala, P.K. Moore

Department of Pharmacology, Cardiovascular Biology Group, National University of Singapore, Singapore

Introduction: Hydrogen sulfide (H_2S) is a naturally occurring gas, which has been shown to be a potent vasodilator. Cystathionine-γ-lyase (CSE) is the key enzyme that utilizes L-cysteine as a substrate to form H_2S in the cardiovascular system. A potential role of H_2S in an inflammatory condition, such as acute pancreatitis and associated lung injury has, however, not been previously described.

Methods: Acute pancreatitis was induced in mice by hourly intraperitoneal injections of caerulein. Presence of CSE mRNA in the pancreas was determined by RT-PCR. DL-propargylglycine (PAG), is an irreversible inhibitor of CSE, was administered (100 mg/kg i.p.) either one hour before or one hour after starting caerulein injections and pancreatic inflammation and lung injury were assessed.

Results: We found the presence of H_2S synthesizing enzyme activity and CSE (as determined by mRNA signal) in the pancreas. Also, prophylactic, as well as therapeutic, treatment with PAG, significantly reduced the severity of caerulein-induced pancreatitis and associated lung injury, as determined by 1) hyperamylasemia [plasma amylase (U/L) (control, 1204 $\pm$ 59); prophylactic treatment: placebo, 10635 $\pm$ 305; PAG, 7904 $\pm$ 495; therapeutic treatment: placebo, 10427 $\pm$ 470; PAG, 7811 $\pm$ 428; $p < 0.05$ PAG c.f. placebo; $n = 24$ animals in each group], 2) neutrophil sequestration in the pancreas [pancreatic myeloperoxidase oxidase (MPO) activity (fold increase over control) (prophylactic treatment: placebo, 5.78 $\pm$ 0.63; PAG, 2.97 $\pm$ 0.39; therapeutic treatment: placebo, 5.48 $\pm$ 0.52; PAG, 3.03 $\pm$ 0.47; $p < 0.05$ PAG c.f. placebo; $n = 24$ animals in each group)], 3) pancreatic acinar cell injury/necrosis, 4) lung MPO activity (fold increase over control) [prophylactic treatment: placebo, 1.99 $\pm$ 0.16; PAG, 1.34 $\pm$ 0.14; therapeutic treatment: placebo, 2.03 $\pm$ 0.12; PAG, 1.41 $\pm$ 0.97; $p < 0.05$ PAG c.f. placebo; $n = 24$ animals in each group] and 5) histological evidence of lung injury.

Conclusions: These results suggest an important proinflammatory role for H_2S in the pathogenesis of acute pancreatitis and associated lung injury.

33

Treatment with Bindarit, a Blocker of MCP-1 Synthesis, Protects Mice Against Acute Pancreatitis

M. Bhatia[1], R.D. Ramnath[1], L. Chevali[1], A. Guglielmotti[2]

[1]Department of Pharmacology, National University of Singapore, Singapore; [2]ACRAF SpA, S.Palomba-Pomezia, Rome, Italy

Introduction: Chemokines are believed to play a key role in the pathogenesis of acute pancreatitis. We have earlier shown that pancreatic acinar cells produce the chemokine MCP-1 in response to caerulein hyperstimulation, demonstrating that acinar-derived MCP-1 is an early mediator of inflammation in acute pancreatitis. Blocking chemokine production or action is a major target for pharmacological intervention in a variety of inflammatory diseases, such as acute pancreatitis. Bindarit (2-methyl-2-[[1-(phenylmethyl)-1H-indazol-3yl]methoxy]propanoic acid) has been shown to preferentially inhibit MCP-1 production in vitro in monocytes and in vivo, without affecting the production of the cytokines IL-1, IL-6, or the chemokines IL-8, MIP-1α and RANTES. The present study aimed to define the role of MCP-1 in acute pancreatitis by the use of bindarit.

Methods: Acute pancreatitis was induced in mice by hourly intraperitoneal injections of caerulein. Bindarit was administered either one hour before or one hour after starting caerulein injections and the severity of acute pancreatitis was assessed. MCP-1 levels were determined by ELISA.

Results: Prophylactic as well as therapeutic treatment with bindarit significantly reduced MCP-1 levels in the pancreas. Also, this treatment significantly protected mice against acute pancreatitis as determined by hyperamylasemia, neutrophil sequestration in the pancreas (pancreatic MPO activity), and pancreatic acinar cell injury/necrosis on histological examination of pancreas sections.

Conclusions: These results show an important role of MCP-1 in the pathogenesis of acute pancreatitis and suggest that anti MCP-1 strategies may be of potential therapeutic value in the treatment of acute pancreatitis.

34

n-3, n-6 and n-9 Polyunsaturated Fatty Acids – Which Composition in Parenteral Nutrition Decreases Severity of Acute Hemorrhagic Necrotizing Pancreatitis in Rats?

F.A. Wenger[1], M. Kilian[2], I. Heukamp[3], J.I. Gregor[2], M. Hanel[2], I. Schimke[4], H. Guski[5], M.K. Walz[1], J.M. Müller[2]

[1]Clinic of Surgery and Centre of Minimal-invasive Surgery, Ev. Huyssens-Stiftung und Knappschafts-GmbH, Kliniken Essen-Mitte, Essen, [2]Clinic of General, Visceral, Vascular and Thoracic Surgery, [3]Clinic of Internal Medicine IV, [4]Clinic of Internal Medicine I, and [5]Institute of Pathology, University Hospital Charité Campus Mitte, Humboldt-University Berlin, Germany

Introduction: Acute pancreatitis often requires parenteral nutrition. Thus we analyzed in a randomized trial whether different fatty acids in parenteral nutrition influence lipid peroxidation and histopathology in acute pancreatitis in rats.

Methods: 75 male Sprague-Dawley rats were randomized into 5 groups (gr.) (n = 15). Gr. 1 underwent a laparotomy followed by saline infusion, gr. 2–5 received intraductal GDOC followed by intravenous cerulein. 6 hours after induction of pancreatitis (IOP) gr. 3 received a standard lipovenous infusion (rich in [n–6] polyunsaturated fatty acids (PUFA)), gr. 4 was infused ClinOleic (rich in [n-9] PUFA) while gr. 5 received infusion of Omegaven (rich in [n-3] PUFA) for 18 hours.

Results: Omegaven infusion reduced severity of histopathologic changes in acute pancreatitis and decreased lipid peroxidation in pancreatic tissue samples. Furthermore lipid production protective enzyme superoxide dismutase (SOD) was increased. However, standard PUFA and ClinOleic infusion did not influence severity of pancreatitis and lipid peroxidation.

Conclusion: Parenteral nutrition high in n-3 PUFA seems to be superior to compositions of n-6 or n-9 PUFA in the treatment of acute hemorrhagic pancreatitis in rats.

35

Combined Intravenous and Oral Selenium Treatment in DBTC-Induced Acute Pancreatitis

J. Merkord[1], N. Görl[1], M. Lembke[1], H. Weber[2], A. Berg[1], G. Hennighausen[1]

[1]Institute of Toxicology, [2]Institute of Pathobiochemistry, University of Rostock, Germany

Introduction: Oxidative stress is one of the mechanisms of propagation of acinar cell injury in acute pancreatitis. Selenium is an essential cofactor in the antioxidant glutathione peroxidase pathway. Serum selenium levels are described to be subnormal in patients with acute and chronic pancreatitis. The present study tests the hypothesis that an bolus of intravenous Na-selenite and the daily oral application of Na-selenite reduce the acute DBTC-pancreatitis in rats.

Methods: Male Lewis rats were randomly allocated to one of 3 groups (n = 6/group) as follows: Group 1: Na-selenite 5 mg/kg^2 b.w. i.v. and daily Na-selenite 1 mg/kg^2 b.w. p.o.; Group 2: Single dose of 6 mg/kg^2 DBTC i.v.; Group 3: DBTC + Na-selenite (5 mg/kg^2 b.w. i.v. 10 min after DBTC application + daily Na-selenite 1 mg/kg^2 b.w. p.o.). The animals were sacrificed after 4 and 7 days. Follow parameters were studied: malon-dialdehyd (MDA) in serum, amylase and lipase activity in serum, histology of pancreas and the concentration of tin and selenium in pancreas, serum, bile and urine.

Results: In the DBTC group MDA, amylase and lipase in serum were increased. Na-selenite lowered significantly these parameters (MDA after 2 h, amylase and lipase after 24 to 48 h) and the histological signs of pancreatitis (edema, neutrophil infiltration and acinar cell degranulation). Selenium had no effects on tin distribution and elimination. Na-selenite alone (group 1) had no effect on all parameters.

Conclusion: Combined selenium treatment diminished the DBTC-induced pancreatitis in rats. The significant decrease of MDA in serum by selenium is possibly connected with a lower oxidative stress in acute DBTC-pancreatitis.

36

The Effect of Pseudorabies Virus Infection on Pancreatic Duct Cell Secretion

V. Venglovecz[1], Z. Rakonczay Jr.[2,1], B. Ordog[3], T. Takács[1], J. Lonovics[1], A. Szabolcs[1], A. Varro[4], A. Toth[4], J.G. Papp[4], M.A. Gray[2], B.E. Argent[2], Z. Boldogkoi[3], P. Hegyi[1,2]

[1]First Department of Medicine Faculty of Medicine, University of Szeged, Szeged, Hungary; [2]School of Cell & Molecular Biosciences, University Medical School, Newcastle upon Tyne, UK; [3]Department of Biology, Faculty of Medicine, University of Szeged, Hungary, [4]Department of Pharmacology and Pharmacotherapy, Faculty of Medicine, Division of Cardiovascular Pharmacology, Hungarian Academy of Sciences, University of Szeged, Hungary

Background: We have previously shown that hypersecretion can be observed during the early phase of experimental oedematous and necrotizing pancreatitis. However, the source and the role of hypersecretion are unknown. Several viruses have been reported to cause acute pancreatitis, but we have no information concerning the effect of viral infection on pancreatic secretion. Our aim in this study was to examine the effect of acute infection caused by a herpes virus (pseudorabies virus; PRV) on pancreatic ductal secretion.

Methods: Ba-DupGreen (BDG), a genetically modified replicating strain of PRV was used in this study. The green fluorescent protein (GFP) gene was inserted into the PRV antisense promoter region located in the inverted repeat segment of the virus. Small intra/interlobular ducts were isolated from the pancreas of guinea pigs. Ducts were incubated in McCoy's based culture medium containing BDG virus (10^7 plaque forming units/ml) for 6 hours, while the control ducts were incubated only with the culture media. The ducts were then cultured for further 18 hours. The rate of HCO_3^- secretion was determined as described earlier (Hegyi et al. Am J Physiol Cell Physiol 2003;285:C268–C276). All the experiments were performed in HCO_3^--buffered Ringer solution at 37°C. Viral structural proteins were visualized by immunohistochemistry. Native GFP expression and immunofluorescence signals were recorded by a confocal laser scanning microscope.

Results and Conclusions: The virus infected all accessible epithelial cells of the duct as judged by the appearance of GFP and viral antigens in the ductal cells. PRV infection stimulated ductal HCO_3^- secretion about 4–5-fold after 24 h. We suggest that this response of pancreatic ducts to PRV infection could represent a defence mechanism against invasive pathogens to avoid pancreatic injury.

This work was supported by The Wellcome Trust and OTKA.

37

Pro- and Anti-Inflammatory Response of Acinar Cells to Pancreatitis-Associated Ascitic Fluid during Experimental Acute Pancreatitis

L. Ramudo[1], M.A. Manso[1], S. Vicente[2], R. Rodriguez[1], A. Garcia-Montero[1], I. De Dios[1]

[1]Department of Physiology and Pharmacology, and [2]Department of Toxicology, University of Salamanca, Spain

Introduction and Aims: Acute pancreatitis (AP) is associated with increased cytokine release from different cell sources. A delicate balance between pro- and anti-inflammatory mediators determines the nature of the inflammatory response. We investigate the ability of acinar cells to produce tumor necrosis factor α (TNF-α) and interleukin-10 (IL-10) in response to pancreatitis-associated ascitic fluid (PAAF) at different AP stages.

Methods: AP was induced in rats by bile-pancreatic duct obstruction (BPDO). Acinar cells resuspended in culture medium containing brefeldin A were incubated for 4 h in 5% CO2 atmosphere at 37°C in absence and presence of 24-h BPDO-PAAF (20% v/v). Analysis of the acinar TNF-α and IL-10 production was carried out by flow cytometry using phycoerythrin-labelled monoclonal antibodies.

Results: Acinar cells of control rats demonstrated an ability to produce and IL-10 in response to PAAF. TNF-α production was also stimulated by PAAF in rats with AP; however, the pro-inflammatory response was found significantly ($p < 0.05$) reduced from 6 h after BPDO. On the other hand, acinar cells failed to produce IL-10 in response to PAAF from 3 h after BPDO. A detailed analysis of cytokine production in the two acinar cell populations (R1 and R2) differentiated by flow cytometry on the basis of the forward scatter (FSC), revealed greater ($p < 0.05$) ability in R2 cells to produce TNF-α and IL-10 in response to PAAF. From 6 h after BPDO no differential behaviour was found between either cell subsets.

Conclusions: 1) PAAF stimulates the acinar production of TNF-α not IL-10 during AP. 2) The balance between the acinar production of pro- and anti-inflammatory cytokines is increased from early AP stages. 3) Acinar cells with higher FSC display a greater ability to produce cytokines up to 6 h after BPDO.

Supported by FIS (PI02/163) and Junta Castilla León (SA123/03), Spain.

38

Protective Effect of Ghrelin in Ischemia/Reperfusion-Induced Acute Pancreatitis in Rats

Z. Warzecha[1], A. Dembiński[1], J. Jaworek[1], W.W. Pawlik[1], R. Tomaszewska[2], B. Kuśnierz-Cabala[3], J.W. Naskalski[3], P.C. Konturek[4], A. Kuwahara[5], I. Kato[6]

[1]Department of Physiology, [2]Department of Pathology and [3]Department of Clinical Biochemistry, Jagiellonian University Medical College, Krakow, Poland; [4]Department of Internal Medicine I, University of Erlangen-Nuremberg, Erlangen, Germany; [5]Institute for Environmental Sciences, University of Shizuoka, Japan, [6]Yanaihara Institute Inc., Shizuoka, Japan

Background: Ghrelin, an endogenous ligand for the growth hormone secretagogue receptor, was primary isolated from the human and rat stomach. It stimulates growth hormone secretion, food intake and exhibits gastroprotective properties. In the previous study, we have found the protective effect of ghrelin against edematous caerulein-induced pancreatitis. The aim of present study was to investigate the influence of ghrelin administration on the development of acute hemorrhagic pancreatitis.

Methods: Acute pancreatitis was induced in rat by clamping of inferior splenic artery for 30 min followed by reperfusion. Ghrelin was administered twice (30 min prior to start of ischemia and after next 3 h) at the doses: 4, 8 or 16 nmol/kg/dose. After 6-h reperfusion animals were sacrificed and the following parameters were measured: pancreatic blood flow, pancreatic DNA synthesis, serum lipase and poly-C ribonuclease activity, serum interleukin-1 (IL-1), interleukin-10 (IL-10), growth hormone (GH) and insulin-like growth factor-1 (IGF-1) concentration and morphological signs of pancreatitis.

Results: Treatment with ghrelin attenuated the development of ischemia/reperfusion-induced pancreatitis, what was demonstrated in histological examination as the reduction in pancreatic edema, inflammatory infiltration, necrosis, hemorrhages and the decrease in vacuolization of pancreatic acinar cells. Also, ghrelin administration decreased the activity of lipase and poly-C ribonuclease, and concentration of pro-inflammatory IL-1 in the serum, whereas the pancreatitis-evoked fall in pancreatic DNA synthesis was partly reversed. Treatment with ghrelin was without effect on the pancreatitis-related fall of pancreatic blood flow. Ischemia/reperfusion-induced pancreatitis strongly reduced serum concentration of GH and IGF-1, and ghrelin administration reversed this effect. Ghrelin at the dose 8 nmol/kg exhibited maximal beneficial effect.

Conclusions: (1) Administration of ghrelin attenuates pancreatic damage in ischemia/reperfusion-induced pancreatitis; (2) Protective effect of ghrelin administration seems to be related to reduction in the release of pro-inflammatory IL-1 and restoration of IGF-1 level to control value.

39

Overexpression of Smad6 in the Pancreatic Acini Alters Actin Dynamics and Inhibits Enzyme Exocytosis

M. Kaku, M. Tashiro, H. Nakamura, M. Otsuki

Department of Gastroenterology and Metabolism, University of Occupational Environmental Health, School of Medicine, Kitakyushu, Fukuoka, Japan

Introduction: Smad6, the inhibitory Smads, is known to inhibit transforming growth factor-β signalings. We had shown that acute pancreatitis induced by intraperitoneal injection of caerulein or by feeding choline-deficient, ethionine-supplemented diet, was aggravated in transgenic mice (Tg) overexpressing Smad6 in the pancreatic acinar cells. To investigate the mechanism for this aggravation of acute pancreatitis in Tg mice, we examined actin dynamics and pancreatic enzyme exocytosis in response to various secretagogues in isolated pancreatic acini.

Method and Results: Pancreatic acini were freshly isolated from Tg mice that overexpress Smad6 specifically in pancreatic acinar cells or control (C57BL/6N) mice by collagenase digestion method. There were no significant differences in pancreatic contents of protein, DNA, amylase and trypsin between Tg and control mice. Amylase secretion in response to 10 pM CCK-8 from Tg mice acini was approximately 30% reduced compared with control mice acini. In Tg mice acini, the responsiveness to carbamylcholine stimulation was also significantly decreased, whereas that to secretin was quite similar to the control. The acini from Tg mice showed a lower responsiveness to fluoride, a potent and direct activator of guanine nucleotide-binding proteins. Filamentous-actin (F-actin) content after stimulation with CCK-8 determined by a rhodamine-conjugated phalloidin binding assay revealed that F-actin content in the isolated acini from Tg mice were similar to the control, but the responsiveness to CCK-8 was considerably reduced.

Conclusion: These results suggest that overexpression of Smad6 decreases exocytosis of digestive enzymes in response to Ca^{2+} mobilizing stimuli due to reduced actin dynamics. Reduction of enzyme exocytosis in Tg mice may contribute to worsen acute pancreatitis.

40

Pancreatic Phospholipase A2 is Activated in the Initial Phase of Experimental Pancreatitis and Contributes to Early Pancreatic Injury

B. Brandt-Nedelev[1], J. Mayerle[2], I. Jaroscakova[1], T. Wartmann[1], H. Lippert[1], D.Y. Hui[3], W. Halangk[1], M.M. Lerch[2]

[1]Division of Experimental Surgery, Otto-von-Guericke-University Magdeburg, Germany, [2]Department of Gastroenterology, Endocrinology and Nutrition, Ernst-Moritz-Arndt-University Greifswald, Germany; [3]Department of Pathology and Laboratory Medicine, University of Cincinnati, OH, USA

Introduction: Digestive zymogens are activated in the pancreatic acinar cell during the early time course of acute pancreatitis. While the activation of proteolytic zymogens was shown in numerous studies, the role of other digestive enzymes is much less clear. In the present study we investigated the role of pancreatic secretory phospholipase A2 (PLA2) in acinar cell injury during an experimental pancreatitis model using PLA2-deficient mice.

Methods: Pancreatic secretory-PLA2-deficient mice were generated by targeted disruption of the PLA2 gene (Gastroenterology 2001;120:1193–1202). Acute pancreatitis was induced by 7 hourly injections of caerulein (50 μg/h, i.p.). Control mice received i.p. saline. Amylase and lipase were enzymatically determined in serum and pancreatic tissue. Pancreatic oedema was calculated as ratio of pancreatic wet weight to body mass. Histological evaluation of pancreatic injury was performed after H&E staining, apoptosis by 3-OH nick-end labelling, and necrosis by EM. Trypsin and cathepsin B were fluorometrically determined.

Results: After supramaximal caerulein stimulation high levels of serum amylase and lipase in wild-type mice indicate early pancreatic injury. In contrast, these enzyme activities were significantly (up to 70%) lower in PLA2−/− mice. This reduction was not due to a lower pancreatic expression of these enzymes in PLA2−/− animals, nor caused by a reduced trypsin or cathepsin B activities (as potentially PLA2-activating enzymes). In later stages of pancreatitis, serum pancreatic enzyme levels and pancreatic oedema developed to comparable levels in both strains of mice. While histological severity and the extent of necrosis was reduced in the PLA2-deficient mice the rate of apoptosis more than doubled.

Conclusion: Our data indicate that the activation of secretory pro-PLA2 is clearly involved in the pathogenesis of acute pancreatitis, and that this enzyme contributes to pancreatic injury by shifting the ratio at which cells die from a predominance of apoptosis to a predominance of necrosis, and thus to greater severitiy.

analysed for haemoglobin and activities of α_1-antitrypsin and α_2-macroglobulin.

Results: Caerulein alone did not induce signs of vascular damage. Tissue haemoglobin levels (6.6 ± 3.9 μg/g dry wt) were similar to those of controls without pancreatitis (3.0 ± 0.6 μg/g). Pretreatment with icatibant produced a significant ($p < 0.01$) elevation in tissue haemoglobin concentrations (31.5 ± 2.9 μg/ml). Although the t-KK inhibitor inhibited oedema formation to an extent similar to icatibant, signs of vascular damage were absent. The haemorrhage induced by icatibant was largely attenuated by a concomitant treatment with FE999024 and FE999026 (12.6 ± 1.3 μg Hb/g). Influx of endogenous inhibitors of kallikreins, α_1-antitrypsin and α_2-macroglobulin, was significantly ($p < 0.05$) reduced by icatibant and FE999024. However, t-KK activity was increased 10–100 fold by icatibant ($p < 0.01$), whereas it was strongly inhibited ($p < 0.05$) by the t-KK inhibitor FE999024.

Conclusions: Our results suggest that de-inhibition of kallikrein activity in the pancreas in the absence of oedema formation is involved in the induction of icatibant-induced haemorrhagic lesions in caerulein-induced pancreatitis. Inhibition of tissue and plasma kallikrein thus seems to be a highly interesting strategy for the prevention of this kind of tissue damage.

41

Peroxisome Proliferator-Activated Receptor-Gamma Agonist Reduces the Severity of Post-ERCP Acute Pancreatitis

D. Closa, S. Granell, E. Folch-Puy

Department of Experimental Pathology, IIBB-CSIC, Barcelona, Spain

Introduction: Acute pancreatitis is a complication of Endoscopic Retrograde CholangioPancreatography (ERCP). Recently, it has been reported that PPAR-gamma agonists reduce the severity of acute pancreatitis induced by cerulein. The aim of this study was to evaluate the effects of prophylactic PPAR-gamma agonist application in an experimental model of post-ERCP acute pancreatitis.

Methods: ERCP-pancreatitis was induced by infusion of contrast medium into the pancreatic duct in male Wistar rats. In the control group, the pancreatic duct was cannulated without infusion. In additional groups, rosiglitazone, a PPAR-gamma agonist, was added to the infusion of contrast medium. 3 h after the intervention, plasma and pancreas samples were obtained and levels of lipase, edema and myeloperoxidase were evaluated.

Results: Infusion of contrast medium into the pancreatic duct resulted in increased lipase levels in plasma, and edema and myeloperoxidase activity in pancreas. Rosiglitazone reduced the increase in lipase and the level of edema and completely abolished the increase in myeloperoxidase.

Conclusions: Prophylactic administration of PPAR-gamma agonist provides a protective effect in experimental post-ERCP pancreatitis. The mechanism of the protective effects of Rosiglitazone seems to be the reduction of leukocyte recruitment.

42

Possible Role of Kallikreins in Haemorrhagic Lesions Induced by a Kinin B$_2$ Receptor Antagonist in Experimental Acute Pancreatitis

T. Griesbacher[1], D.M. Evans[2], B.A. Peskar[1]

[1]Institute for Experimental and Clinical Pharmacology, Medical University of Graz, Austria; [2]Ferring Research Ltd., Southampton, UK

Introduction: Kinin B_2 receptor antagonists effectively prevent oedema formation in experimental caerulein-induced pancreatitis. However, this treatment is accompanied by the formation of haemorrhagic lesions in the pancreas at later time points. We have investigated whether this could be due to the prevention of influx of endogenous protease inhibitors into the pancreas and concomitant augmentation of tissue kallikrein activity.

Methods: Pancreatitis was induced in anaesthetized rats by i.v. infusion of caerulein. Animals were pretreated with the selective B_2 antagonist icatibant and or the selective inhibitors for tissue kallikrein (t-KK) (FE999024) and plasma kallikrein (FE999026). Six h later, pancreatic tissue samples were excised, assessed histologically, and

43

Diverse Roles of Class I PI3K Isoforms δ and γ in Cerulein-Induced Pancreatitis: PI3K δ is Necessary for Trypsinogen Activation

L. Fischer[1,2], A. Lugea[1], J.M. Penninger[3], B. Vanhaesebroeck[4], M.W. Büchler[2], H. Friess[2], A.S. Gukovskaya[1], S.J. Pandol[1], I. Gukovsky[1]

[1]VA Greater Los Angeles Healthcare System & University of California, Los Angeles, CA, USA; [2]University of Heidelberg, Germany; [3]Institute for Molecular Biotechnology, Austrian Academy of Sciences, Vienna, Austria; [4]Ludwig Institute for Cancer Research, London, UK

Background and Aims: Phosphoinositol 3-kinase (PI3K) is a key signaling molecule. Its function in pancreatitis is poorly understood. We sought to determine the roles of inducible PI3K isoforms δ and γ in the cerulein (CR) model of acute pancreatitis.

Methods: To inactivate PI3K we used mice deficient in PI3Kγ catalytic subunit, p110γ, or homozygous for the loss-of-function p110δ ^{D910A} mutant of PI3Kδ. Pancreatitis was induced by up to 7 hourly i.p. injections of CR; controls received saline. We measured both early and late responses of pancreatitis at 30 min and 7 h after the 1st CR injection.

Results: Genetic inactivation of either PI3K δ or γ reduced neutrophil infiltration by ~2-fold. Pancreatic NF-κB activation and necrosis were also inhibited. However, serum amylase and lipase levels, and acinar cell vacuolization were unaffected. PI3K δ or γ inactivation stimulated apoptosis in pancreatitis by up to 2-fold. Caspase-3 activity did not increase, suggesting that PI3K regulates apoptosis via a caspase-independent mechanism. Lysosomal markers, such as hexosaminidase, was inhibited by PI3K δ or γ inactivation by 85 and 65%, respectively. Cathepsin B activity was also inhibited in PI3K mutant mice. These data indicate important roles for both PI3K isoforms in lysosomal activation in CR pancreatitis. In both mutants, trypsinogen activation in pancreatitis was markedly reduced at both early and late time points, with the late phase completely inhibited in PI3Kδ mutant mice. Trypsinogen activation by CR was only partially reduced in pancreatic acini isolated from PI3K δ or γ mutant mice (compared to wild type), suggesting that non-acinar cells may regulate trypsinogen activation in pancreatitis via PI3K. Furthermore, blood neutrophils isolated from both PI3K mutant mice displayed impaired oxidative burst.

Conclusions: PI3K δ and γ isoforms regulate key responses of pancreatitis. The results further elucidate the role of the inflammatory response in pancreatic injury.

44

Activation of Polyamine Catabolism Response to Trypsin Activation in Sodium Taurocholate Pancreatitis Model

H. Jin[1], T. Lämsä[1], K.-H. Herzig[2], J. Sand[1], S. Räty[1], L. Alhonen[2], I. Nordback[1]

[1]Department of Gastroenterology and Alimentary Tract Surgery, Tampere University Hospital, and [2]A.I. Virtanen Institute for Molecular Sciences, University of Kuopio, Finland

Introduction: Polyamine homeostasis is essential for tissue survival and growth. With acute pancreatic inflammation, polyamine catabolism is activated with induction of spermidine/spermine N'-acetyltransferase (SSAT). The aim of this study was to monitor changes in SSAT induction and respective polyamine depletion (spermidine, spermine) with respect to trypsin activation in sodium taurocholate pancreatitis model of rats.

Methods: 60 Sprague-Dawley rats (300 g–350 g) were divided into 2 groups. In pancreatitis group 0.2 ml of 2.0% sodium taurocholate was infused into the pancreatic duct, and in sham group only laparotomy was performed. All animals were sacrificed and sampled under anesthesia at 1.5 h, 3 h, 6 h, 24 h and 48 h. Six rats served as 0 hour controls without operation. Pancreatitis was monitored with pancreatic water content, histology and serum amylase activity. Concentrations of spermidine, spermine and SSAT in the pancreas were analysed. Trypsin activation was measured by analysing pancreatic trypsin activation peptide (TAP) concentration.

Results: Sodium taurocholate infusion induced pancreatitis with hyperamylasemia, pancreatic edema, and pancreatitis histology. Pancreatic SSAT and trypsin activation were induced and they peaked simultaneously (Table), followed by substantial decrease of both spermidine and spermine in the pancreas.

Conclusions: Sodium taurocholate induced experimental pancreatitis is associated with both trypsin activation and simultaneous activation of polyamine catabolism. It remains to be shown whether these phenomenons are coinciding or dependent one on the other.

Table of Abstract 44

Group	Parameters	1.5 hours	3 hours	6 hours	24 hours	48 hours
sham	SSAT (pmol/mg prot./10 min)	10.6 ± 2.7	83.9 ± 21.4	38.7 ± 5.6	74.8 ± 7.3	74.1 ± 17.4
	TAP (pmol/mg prot.)	10.1 ± 2.4	9.6 ± 3.4	8.1 ± 1.5	10.1 ± 2.2	4.4 ± 0.7
	SPD (pmol/mg prot.)	22.3 ± 0.9	29.8 ± 0.4	23.4 ± 0.5	25.2 ± 1.7	24.9 ± 4.9
	SPM (pmol/mg prot.)	3.9 ± 0.3	3.9 ± 0.2	3.8 ± 0.1	3.7 ± 0.3	3.7 ± 0.6
AP	SSAT (pmol/mg prot./10 min)	17.3 ± 6.7	563.9 ± 137.6 *	343.8 ± 16.5 *	190.3 ± 63.3	47.3 ± 8.8
	TAP (pmol/mg prot.)	9.2 ± 3.1	71.6 ± 11.0 *	14.4 ± 3.6	25.4 ± 4.7 *	9.0 ± 4.3
	SPD (pmol/mg prot.)	25.8 ± 1.5	20.5 ± 3.8 *	24.6 ± 0.5	11.8 ± 3.0 *	29.6 ± 3.9
	SPM (pmol/mg prot.)	3.8 ± 0.2	3.4 ± 0.3	4.1 ± 0.2	2.8 ± 0.2 *	4.1 ± 0.6

SPD: spermidine; SPM: spermine; AP: acute pancreatitis. Compared to sham group (means ± SE), *$p < 0.05$.

45

The Expression of Vacuole Membrane Protein 1 (VMP1) Induces Autophagic Process in Pancreatic Acinar Cells

M.I. Vaccaro[1], D. Grasso[1], R. Pardo[1], A. Ropolo[1], C.D. Gonzalez[1], J.L. Iovanna[2]

[1]School of Medicine, Buenos Aires University, Buenos Aires, Argentina; [2]Unité 624, INSERM, Marseille, France

Introduction: Autophagy is a mechanism that maintains cell survival through the catabolism of its own structure. Intracellular vacuole formation has been reported as an early acinar cell event during acute pancreatitis. We have previously characterized a novel membrane protein, named VMP1, which is induced in acinar cells early during pancreatitis, its expression correlates with vacuole formation and precedes cell death. In order to know the role of VMP1 expression, we tested the hypothesis that VMP1 promotes autophagic process in pancreatic acinar cells.

Methods: Autophagic processes were assayed using AR4-2J pancreatic acinar cells. Polyclonal rabbit antibody was developed using a VMP1-specific peptide antigen. VMP1/V5 and VMP1/EGFP expression plasmids and VMP-RNAi were constructed.

Results: Electron microscopy studies showed that VMP1-induced vacuoles have ultrastructural features of autophagy. Autophagosomes, a double membrane structure containing undigested cytoplasmic material including organelles, as well as autolysosomes, single membrane structure containing cytoplasmic components at various stages of degradation, were observed in VMP1 expressing cells. VMP1-induced vacuoles stained with monodansylcadaverine, a fluorescent tracer for autophagic vacuoles. LC3, a specific marker for autophagic membranes, co-localizes with VMP1 in VMP1/EGFP and VMP1/V5 transfected cells. These results strongly suggest that VMP1 expression induces autophagic vacuoles in pancreatic acinar cells. In other series of experiments, AR4-2J cells were treated with rapamycin, a drug that induces autophagy, and VMP1 over-expression was demonstrated by RT-PCR and Western blot analysis. Immunofluorescence and immunoelectron microscopy of VMP1 in rapamycin-treated cells confirmed that VMP1 is located in autophagic vacuoles. Finally, RNAi silencing of VMP1 expression prevents autophagy induced by rapamycin demonstrating that VMP1 expression is required to the autophagic process.

Conclusions: Our results demonstrate that VMP1 expression promotes autophagy in acinar cells. We propose that the early expression of VMP1 during acute pancreatitis may induce an autophagic process which can protect acinar cells from death.

46

Enalapril Increases the Local Extravasation of Macromolecules and Nitric Oxide Synthase in Pancreas of the Fructose-Fed Insulin Resistant Rat Model

L. Bouffard, M.-O. Hogue, P. St-Pierre, M.-E. Papirakis, P. Maheux

Division of Endocrinology and Metabolism, Department of Medicine, Université de Sherbrooke, Québec, Canada

Introduction: Angiotensin-converting enzyme inhibitors (ACEI) have been associated with an increase risk of acute pancreatitis. Although the pathogenesis is still unclear, an activation of the kinin system and consequently a localized angioedema are thought to lead to acute pancreatic damage. The goal of the present study was to explore the impact of ACEI on pancreatic microcirculation and capillary permeability in normal and insulin resistant rats.

Methods: Chow- and fructose-fed Sprague-Dawley rats were treated with enalapril (10 mg/kg/d) or the vehicle only for 4 weeks before measuring in vivo the extravasation of Evans Blue (EB) dye in pancreas specifically. Unanaesthetized animals (10–15/group) were injected with EB 20 mg/kg in the caudal vein 10 min before sacrifice and EB dye was extracted by formamide from each pancreas.

Results: Relative to controls, enalapril-treated animals showed a very important increase in pancreatic extravasation of EB ($\Delta = +409\%$; $p < 0.001$) in the fructose-fed rat model, while no changes were observed in the chow-fed animals treated with enalapril. In the fructose-fed rats treated with enalapril, serum amylase concentrations were not increased compared to controls; nor was there any difference in total plasma nitrites/nitrates concentrations. This increase in pancreatic vasopermeability seen with enalapril in the fructose-fed animals was accompanied by a significant increase in total pancreatic nitric oxide synthase (NOS) activity compared to controls ($\Delta = +125\%$; $p < 0.001$). This increase in NOS activity seemed to be solely attributable to an upregulation of the endothelial NOS isoform as only the eNOS immunoreactive mass (as opposed to nNOS or iNOS) appeared to be increased in the pancreas of these animals.

Conclusions: Enalapril increases capillary permeability (extravasation of macromolecules) in the pancreas of the fructose-fed rat model. This suggests that ACEI upregulates the eNOS isoform locally, increases vasopermeability of the pancreas and can therefore result in local edema in the fructose-fed insulin resistant rat model.

47

CGRP Enhances MAP Kinase Activation Induced by CCK Stimulation in Rat Pancreatic Lobules

Y. Matsuhashi[1], Y. Tando[1], Y. Ogawa[1], T. Nakamura[2]

[1]Third Department of Internal Medicine, [2]Healthcare Unit, Hirosaki University School of Medicine, Hirosaki, Japan

Introduction: In the early phase of acute pancreatitis, intracellular inflammation-related signals such as NF-κB are activated. Calcitonin gene-related peptide (CGRP) is one of the vasodilative peptides which regulates microcirculation. It is recognized that CGRP attenuates organic damages including pancreas, but it is unclear whether CGRP directly affects on the pancreatic lobules or not. We investigated the direct action of CGRP on the intracellular inflammation-related signals in the pancreatic lobules.

Methods: Pancreas was removed from male Wister rats under ether anesthesia. Minced pancreatic lobules were incubated with either CGRP or cholecystokinin (CCK) or both. Pancreatic lobules were homogenized and the homogenates were analysed in the following examinations. The degradation of IκBα, the phosphorylation of extracellular regulated kinase (ERK), c-Jun N-terminal kinase (JNK) and p38 mitogen-activated protein (MAP) kinases were assessed by western blot analysis. Homogenated pancreatic lobules were ultracentrifuged and the mitochondrial release of cytochrome c into cytosolic fraction was detected by western blot analysis. NF-κB activation was estimated by ELISA.

Results: The cytoplasmic IκBα levels were reduced by CCK stimulation, but CGRP didn't affect the reduction by CCK stimulation. ERK and p38 MAP kinases were phosphorylated by CGRP stimulation, and CGRP enhanced the phosphorylation of MAP kinases by CCK stimulation. CCK activated NF-κB in time-dependent manner, but CGRP didn't activate.

Conclusions: Our results indicated that CGRP directly affected on the phosphorylation of MAP kinases in pancreatic lobules without functioning NF-κB signals. Further investigation are needed to see if this function of CGRP is associated with organ protection.

48

Effects of Calcium on Zymogen Activation in Mouse Pancreatic Acinar Cells

R.D. Smith[1], M. Raraty[2], D.N. Criddle[1], O.V. Gerasimenko[1], A.V. Tepikin[1], J.P. Neoptolemos[2], O.H. Petersen[1], R. Sutton[2]

[1]MRC Secretory Control Research Group, Department of Physiology, and [2]Division of Surgery and Oncology, University of Liverpool, UK

Introduction: Pancreatic digestive proenzymes are condensed in an inactive form within zymogen granules by high concentrations of calcium, released in response to second messengers and partially replaced by potassium during exocytosis, assisting in enzyme solubilisation. We hypothesize that premature enzyme activation, characteristic of acute pancreatitis, occurs within zymogen granules because of excessive granular calcium depletion, through calcium-induced granular calcium release from abnormal, prolonged cytosolic calcium ($[Ca^{2+}]_i$). We investigated the effects of abnormal calcium signalling on granular enzyme activity.

Methods: Pancreatic acinar cells were isolated from CD1 mice and zymogen granules prepared by the method of Gerasimenko et al. (Cell 1996;84:473–480). Prolonged, abnormal elevations of $[Ca^{2+}]_i$ were induced in cells using 10 nM cholecystokinin (CCK) or 2 μM thapsigargin (TG), whilst isolated granular calcium was depleted by application of 1 mM EGTA and 20 μM ionomycin. Trypsin activity or cathepsin B activity were measured using the fluorescent probes IPR-CMAC or $(FR)_2$-R110 respectively.

Results: Prolonged, abnormal elevation of $[Ca^{2+}]_i$ following CCK or TG, induced trypsinogen activation within 300 s, detected by CMAC fluorescence in rounded compartments up to 1 μm diameter throughout the granular pole of the cell. Similar changes occurred in R110 fluorescence indicating cathepsin B activity, but no increase in the activity of either enzyme was observed in cells preloaded with the calcium chelator BAPTA. In IPR-CMAC loaded isolated granules, decreasing intra-granular calcium resulted in an increase in fluorescence (44 ± 9 a.u.; n = 10) that was inhibited by a protease inhibitor cocktail (98.9 ± 0.1% inhibition; n = 20) or by the specific trypsin inhibitor benzamidine (n = 12). Decreasing granular calcium also increased cathepsin B activity.

Conclusion: These results suggest that premature pancreatic digestive enzyme activation occurs within zymogen granules following granular calcium depletion, consistent with calcium-induced calcium release through excessive acinar $[Ca^{2+}]_i$.

This work was supported by the Medical Research Council UK.

49

Bile Sensitises Inositol Trisphosphate and Ryanodine Receptors to Excessive Calcium Release in Mouse Pancreatic Acinar Cells

J.A. Murphy[1,2], D.N. Criddle[1], M. Raraty[2], J.P. Neoptolemos[2], A.V. Tepikin[1], O.H. Petersen[1], R. Sutton[2]

MRC Secretory Control Research Group, [1]The Physiology Laboratory and [2]Division of Surgery and Oncology, University of Liverpool, UK

Introduction: Abnormal sustained intracellular calcium elevation is implicated in premature intracellular digestive enzyme activation, NF-kappa B activation and subsequent acute pancreatitis. We have shown that naturally occurring bile salts produce pathological calcium elevations (global cytosolic calcium elevations lasting longer than 30 seconds), and have now evaluated whether the second messengers inositol trisphosphate (IP_3), nicotinic adenine acid dinucleotide phosphate (NAADP), cyclic-ADP-ribose (cADPr) and their receptors are integral to this process.

Methods: Isolated mouse pancreatic acinar cells were loaded with a calcium-sensitive dye (Fluo 4) and examined by confocal microscopy (Zeiss LSM510) with excitation at 488 nm and emission collected through a LP 505 nm filter. IP_3, NAADP and cADPr were applied internally via a patch pipette, and taurolithocholic-3-sulphate (TLCS) was perfused extracellularly (10 μM, a concentration below that inducing pathological calcium elevations) and whole-cell voltage clamp recordings made.

Results: Physiological concentrations of IP_3 (1–2 μM) induced typical transient currents and localised calcium spiking in the apical granular pole of the acinar cell. Perfusion of TLCS (10 μM) outside the cell transformed this response into pathological calcium elevations (16 of 18 cells) that were prevented by caffeine (20 mM), an IP_3 receptor antagonist. In contrast, NAADP (50 nM) induced calcium spiking that was not affected by the addition of TLCS (8 of 9 cells). Typical physiological calcium signalling induced by cADPr (10–15 μM) was also transformed into pathological calcium elevation by TLCS (10 μM; 12 of 14 cells).

Conclusions: Physiological calcium signals induced by IP_3 and cADPr are transformed into pathological global cytosolic calcium elevations by low concentrations of the bile salt TLCS. This effect is mediated by altered sensitivity of IP_3 and cADPr receptors, which are potential therapeutic targets.

Acknowledgements

This work was supported by the Medical Research Council, UK. J.M. was supported by CORE through an Amelie Waring Fellowship.

50

The Effect of Resveratrol on Cholecystokinin Octapeptide-Induced Experimental Pancreatitis in Rats

A. Szabolcs[1], T. Takács[1], I. Varga[2], Cs. Varga[3], A. Berkó[3], J. Kaszaki[4], T. Letoha[5], L.Tiszlavicz[6], R. Sári[1], J. Lonovics[1]

[1]First Department of Medicine, Faculty of Medicine, [2]Biological Isotope Laboratory, [3]Department of Comparative Physiology, [4]Institute of Experimental Surgery, [5]Institute of Chemisty, [6]Department of Pathology, University of Szeged, Hungary

Introduction: Resveratrol is a phytoalexin found in the skin of grapes and in red wine. The antioxidant, anti-inflammatory and anticancer effects of the substance were shown in several in vivo and in vitro experiments. This dietary component is thought to be responsible for the so-called 'French paradox', describing the association of red wine consumption and reduced mortality of breast cancer and coronary heart disease. The aim of this study was to test the effect of resveratrol on the cholecystokinin-octapeptide (CCK-8) induced acute pancreatitis model in rats.

Methods: Male Wistar rats were divided into three groups (n = 5 in each). In group C acute pancreatitis was induced by three subcutaneous injections of 75 μg/kg CCK-8 at intervals of 1 h. Rats in group RC received a single dose of 10 mg/kg body weight resveratrol i.p. 30 min prior to CCK-8. Rats in group PS served as control animals and received injections of physiological saline. Animals were sacrificed 4 h after the last CCK-8 injection.

Results: Administration of CCK-8 resulted in significant elevation of the pancreatic weight/bodyweight ratio, serum amylase and lipase activities, whereas the serum glucose, calcium, ASAT and creatinin levels decreased significantly. The development of an edematous pancreatitis was confirmed by histology. In group RC resveratrol significantly reduced the CCK-8-induced changes of all laboratory parameters, and reduced the edema and acinar vacuolisation in the pancreas vs. group C. The activities of free-radical scavenger enzymes and cNOS decreased significantly in the pancreas in group C and RC vs. group PS. In the liver, administration of resveratrol significantly increased the amount of reduced glutathion vs. group PS, and prevented the significant reduction of catalase activity.

Conclusion: Our results demonstrate the beneficial effect of resveratrol on the laboratory and histological parameters of CCK-8-induced acute pancreatitis.

Supported by the Hungarian Scientific Research Fund (T042589).

51

Calcium-Induced Toxicity of Non-Oxidative Ethanol Metabolites in Mouse Pancreatic Acinar Cells: Involvement of ER Calcium Stores and Mitochondrial Function

D.N. Criddle[1], G. Fistetto[1], A.V. Tepikin[1], J.P. Neoptolemos[2], O.H. Petersen[1], R. Sutton[2]

Medical Research Council Secretory Control Research Group, Departments of [1]Physiology and [2]Surgery, University of Liverpool, UK

Background and Aims: Fatty acid ethyl esters (FAEEs) are non-oxidative ethanol metabolites that cause pancreatic acinar cell damage by inducing sustained elevations of the cytosolic Ca^{2+} concentration ($[Ca^{2+}]$). We sought to determine the mechanisms of cytosolic $[Ca^{2+}]$ elevation induced by FAEE.

Methods: Isolated mouse pancreatic acinar cells were loaded with fluorescent dyes to measure by confocal microscopy changes, induced by palmitoleic acid ethyl ester (POAEE) or palmitoleic acid (POA), in $[Ca^{2+}]$ in the cytosol (Fluo 4, Fura Red), and in the endoplasmic reticulum (ER) (Mg Fluo 4), as well as mitochondrial membrane potential (TMRM) and NADH production (autofluorescence). Whole-cell patch-clamp was used to measure Ca^{2+}-dependent currents and apply ethanol metabolites, ATP and/or Ca^{2+} signalling receptor antagonists intracellularly.

Results: Patch-pipette application of POAEE (100 μM) but not POA (50 and 100 μM) induced transient, oscillatory increases of cytosolic $[Ca^{2+}]$ and Ca^{2+}-dependent currents prevented by caffeine (20 mM), but not atropine nor ryanodine, indicating mediation by inositol trisphosphate receptors (IP_3R). Extracellular POAEE (100 μM) or POA (50 μM) induced ER Ca^{2+} release that was not prevented by caffeine, ryanodine or atropine. With extracellular Ca^{2+}, cytosolic Ca^{2+} accumulated, suggesting Ca^{2+}-ATPase pump failure. This caused cell blebbing and subsequent lysis. Both metabolites decreased NADH autofluorescence, indicating inhibition of mitochondrial metabolism. Mitochondrial depolarisation was induced by 100 μM POAEE or 50 μM POA, accompanied by a sustained rise of cytosolic $[Ca^{2+}]$, but not 10 μM POA, despite a sustained but smaller rise in cytosolic $[Ca^{2+}]$. Patch-pipette application of ATP abolished the sustained rise in cytosolic $[Ca^{2+}]$ in response to both POAEE and POA, although with POAEE transient oscillatory signals persisted that were prevented by caffeine.

Conclusions: FAEEs increase cytosolic $[Ca^{2+}]$ via ER Ca^{2+} release through IP_3Rs and Ca^{2+}-ATPase pump failure caused by insufficient mitochondrial ATP production, an important determinant of pancreatic cellular toxicity.

Acknowledgement

This work was supported by the Medical Research Council, UK.

52

Severe Acute Pancreatitis Induces a State of Diminished Responsiveness to Lipopolysaccharide

D.J. Mole[1], N.V. McFerran[2], T. Diamond[1]

[1]Surgery, School of Medicine and [2]Biology and Biochemistry, Queen's University of Belfast, Northern Ireland

Introduction: The extent of the role of lipopolysaccharide (LPS) during systemic inflammation in severe acute pancreatitis (AP) is unclear. Kumar has recently shown that diminished responsiveness to LPS, similar to that induced by classical endotoxin tolerance may be replicated by administration of IL-10. This study tested the hypothesis that the complex inflammatory processes observed during severe AP may induce diminished responsiveness to a delayed 'second hit' of intra-arterial LPS.

Methods: With ethical approval, AP was induced in rats by co-administering intraductal glycodeoxycholic acid and intravenous caerulein. In a $3 \times 2 \times 2$ cubic factorial design, the effect of zero, 6 and 30 μg/kg LPS was measured 30 and 90 minutes after intra-arterial injection, 18 hours after induction of AP or sham laparotomy. The production of 16 cytokines and chemokines was measured in serum by multiplex ELISA.

Results: Four patterns of cytokine response were observed. (1) TNF-α, IL-1α, IL-1β, IL-6, IFN-γ, MCP-1, MIP-2α, MIP-3α, RANTES and fractalkine were produced in a dose-dependent and time-dependent fashion in response to LPS. This response was significantly diminished in AP compared to controls ($p < 0.001$, ANOVA). (2) IL-2, IL-4 and GM-CSF levels were undetectable in all groups. (3) CINC-2α and GRO/KC showed dose- and time-dependent production in response to LPS but little or no difference between AP and controls. (4) IL-10 production after zero and 6 μg/kg LPS injection was significantly higher in AP than controls ($p < 0.001$, ANOVA). IL-10 production after 30 μg/kg injection was the same in AP compared to controls.

Conclusions: Severe acute pancreatitis induces a state of diminished responsiveness to an intra-arterial injection of LPS. IL-10 was produced more readily in AP compared to controls in response to low dose LPS. No causal effect of IL-10 was explored. Further investigation is warranted to determine the mechanisms of diminished responsiveness to LPS in AP.

53

CTLA-4, a New Severity Marker for Acute Necrotising Pancreatitis?

J. Mayerle[1], C. Sünder[1], F.-U. Weiss[1], M. Busse[2], K. Eske[1], B.M. Bröker[2], M.M. Lerch[1]

[1]Department of Gastroenterology, Endocrinology and Nutrition, [2]Department of Immunology, Ernst-Moritz-Arndt-University Greifswald, Germany

Introduction: Acute necrotising pancreatitis is characterised by an overwhelming inflammatory immune response syndrome (SIRS). This could be followed by a compensatory anti-inflammatory response syndrome (CARS) which may facilitate infection of the pancreatic necrosis. Since the role, if any, of T cells in acute pancreatitis has not been defined, we have determined the expression of the inhibitory T cell surface molecule CTLA-4 (CD152) in murine models of acute pancreatitis as a marker of T cell involvement.

Methods: Pancreatitis was induced in C57BL6 mice either by 7 hourly injections of caerulein (50 μg/h, i.p.) or retrograde taurocholate (TC) injections into the pancreatic duct (2%, 3% and 4%). All animals were sacrificed after 12 hours. Serum was evaluated for amylase levels and cytokine secretion (TNFα, IFNγ, IL-6, IL-10, IL-12 and MCP-1). Flow cytometry was employed to evaluate T-cell response. Granulocyte infiltration was detected by MPO and staining for GR-1. Apoptosis was detected by direct 3-OH-nick-end-labelling in the thymus. Splenic CTLA-4 expression was either determined by FACS analysis or antibody labelling of cryosections.

Results: TC concentrations of 4% resulted in an overall mortality rate of 85% (50% for 3% TC, 0% for 2% TC), while all caerulein treated animals survived. Pro-inflammatory cytokines, as well as granulocyte activation and tissue infiltration were significantly elevated in taurocholate pancreatitis compared to caerulein pancreatitis. Thymus cell apoptosis was also found to be significantly increased in taurocholate pancreatitis compared to caerulein pancreatitis. Furthermore, we observed a linear correlation of increased CTLA-4 expression to mortality.

Conclusion: We show that, also in mice, retrograde duct injection with taurocholate is a feasible and gradable model of experimental pancreatitis. When compared with a milder model (caerulein) taurocholate-induced pancreatitis involves T-cells suggesting a possible shift from SIRS to CARS as indicated by an increased expression of the inhibitory surface molecule CTLA-4. Further studies will need to clarify whether CTLA-4 could function as a new marker to evaluate severity of acute necrotising pancreatitis.

54

Expression of Transcription Factors Pdx-1, Hnf-1a and Ptf1a, and Cell Proliferation, Are Inversely Regulated after Induction of Acute Experimental Pancreatitis

M.A. Ortiz[1], X. Molero[1], F.X. Real[2], J.R. Malagelada[1]

[1]Digestive System Research Unit, Hospital Universitari Vall d'Hebron, [2]Institut Municipal d'Investigació Mèdica, Barcelona, Spain

Introduction: During organogenesis, terminal differentiation of pancreatic cells is regulated by the sequential expression of a network of transcriptional regulators such as Pdx-1, Hnf-1a and Ptf1a. Their constitutive expression is needed to maintain the specific function of each cell type. In adult individuals regulation of these transcriptional factors may play a key role in tissue repair and regeneration after injury.

Aim: To analyze the expression of Pdx-1, Hnf-1a and Pft1a in acute experimental pancreatitis from onset until full recovery.

Methods: Cerulein pancreatitis was induced in C57BL/6 mice. At timed intervals blood was obtained and pancreases processed for western-blot and immunohistochemistry. Cell proliferation was assessed by Ki67 immunohistochemistry and BrdU uptake.

Results: In normal pancreas Ptf1a is exclusively expressed in acinar cells. Pdx-1 is expressed at high levels in the islets and weakly in some acinar cells. Expression of Hnf-1a is high in the islets and, at a lesser degree, in most acinar cells. Early after pancreatitis nuclear expression of all three transcription factors is greatly diminished. Reexpression is initiated at days 2–4 and progressively increases throughout days 14–20. Fluctuations in Pdx-1 expression always heralds similar changes in Hnf-1a and Ptf1a, and it coincides with the rise and fall of interstitial cell proliferation. Noteworthy, plasma glucose is elevated (245 ± 22 mg/dl) when nuclear Pdx-1 is critically reduced. Expression of Pdx-1 is fully reestablished by day 2, whereas that of Hnf-1a begins at days 3–4 and progressively increases reaching baseline values at days 14–20. Acinar cell proliferation is weakly initiated at day 2, peaks at days 4–7 and decreases to baseline levels by day 14.

Conclusions: Following acute pancreatitis the expression of transcriptional regulators responsible for the terminal differentiation of pancreatic cells is tightly regulated. Their levels of expression are opposed to the reparative proliferation rates of interstitial and acinar cells.

55

Targeted Disruption of Monocyte Chemoattractant Protein-1 (MCP-1) or its Receptor CCR2b in Experimental Acute Pancreatitis: Influence on Local and Systemic Disease Severity

C.M. Krüger, D. Behrendt, B. Glaser, E. Herboth, C. Rubie, M.K. Schilling, B.M. Rau

Department of General- Visceral-, and Vascular Surgery, University of the Saarland, Homburg/Saar, Germany

Introduction: Experimental and clinical studies suggest that chemokines are early mediators of severity in acute pancreatitis (AP). Among the CC-chemokine family we recently observed a dominating role of MCP-1 in this respect (Rau et al. Intensive Care Med 2003; 29:622). To further address this issue we investigated the course of AP in mice with targeted disruption of the MCP-1 gene or the corresponding CCR2b receptor gene.

Materials and Methods: AP was induced in C57BL/6 mice by repeated intraperitoneal (i.p.) injections of cerulein in three experimental groups: 1. wild type C57BL/6 mice (n = 84). 2. mice with targeted disruption of the MCP-1 gene (MCP-1 KO, n = 48), and 3. mice with targeted disruption of the CCR2b gene (CCR2b KO, n = 48). After observation periods of 3, 6, 12, and 24 hours animals were sacrificed and the following parameters were assessed: extent of pancreatic parenchymal necrosis and leukocyte infiltration, pancreatic MCP-1 and CCR2b mRNA expression by real-time PCR, and pancreatic and systemic MCP-1 protein release by ELISAs.

Results: In wild type mice with AP progressive pancreatic parenchymal necrosis and leukocyte infiltration developed within 24 hours. A significant upregulation of intrapancreatic MCP-1 and CCR2b mRNA expression was already present 3 h after induction of AP. Intrapancreatic and systemic MCP-1 protein release revealed a similar course with maximum concentrations at the 12 h interval. Real-time PCR confirmed the absence of MCP-1 and CCR2b mRNA expression in the two knock-out groups. Whereas no relevant pancreatic and systemic MCP-1 protein expression was found in MCP-1 KO mice, concentrations were dramatically increased in CCR2b KO animals throughout the whole experiment. Irrespective of the disrupted gene, the extent intrapancreatic necrosis was not different from wild type mice. However, pancreatic leukocyte tissue infiltration was significantly inhibited in both the MCP-1 and the CCR2b KO group at all time intervals.

Conclusion: AP is associated with an early upregulation of local and systemic MCP-1 concentrations. Our results suggest that binding of MCP-1 to its receptor CCR2b enhances disease severity by promoting leukocyte tissue infiltration and activation.

56

Obese Mice Exhibit an Increased Proinflammatory Response in Cerulein-Induced Pancreatitis

R. Segersvärd[1], J.A. Tsai[1], M.K. Herrington[2], J. Permert[1]

[1]Division of Surgery, Center for Surgical Sciences, Karolinska University Hospital Huddinge, Karolinska Institutet, Stockholm, Sweden; [2]Department of Biology, Adams State College, Alamosa, CO, USA

Introduction: Obesity is associated with an increased severity in human and rat acute pancreatitis (AP), but the underlying mechanisms are not known. The severity of AP is largely determined by a systemic inflammation and involvement of distant organs. In cerulein-induced pancreatitis, the current study evaluated organ injury and gene expression of two pro-inflammatory cytokines, tumor necrosis factor (TNF) and IL-6, and one anti-inflammatory cytokine, IL-10, in the obese ob/ob mice.

Methods: AP was induced in obese and lean mice by 9 hourly injections of cerulein (50 μg/kg i.p.). Saline-injected animals served as controls. Ten hours after the first injection, pancreatic and hepatic injury was assessed by histology, amylase and alanine aminotransferase (ALT). Myeloperoxidase (MPO) activity and gene expression were determined in the pancreas, liver, and lung by real-time PCR.

Results: Obese control mice were hyperglycemic and exhibited severe centrolobular microvesicular steatosis and increased ALT levels compared to lean mice. Obese AP mice had higher amylase levels than the lean AP mice but a similar degree of pancreatic injury and MPO activity. ALT was higher in obese AP mice and they exhibited a more pronounced histological liver pathology. In addition, obese AP mice had a blunted hepatic IL-10 response and increased TNF expression in liver and lung, with a 3-fold higher lung MPO activity compared to lean AP mice ($p = 0.057$).

Conclusion: The obese AP mice exhibited a blunted hepatic anti-inflammatory response, with a concurrent increase in TNF expression and hepatic injury. The increased pulmonary TNF expression and the high lung MPO activity suggest that an increased pulmonary inflammatory response in the obese AP mice. The data also suggest that obesity and hepatic steatosis, perhaps through Kupffer cell dysfunction, increase hepatic injury and augment the inflammatory response, thereby contributing to the enhanced severity of acute pancreatitis seen in obese individuals.

57

Pancreatic Response to Endotoxin after Chronic Alcohol Exposure: Switch from Apoptosis to Necrosis?

F. Fortunato[1], X. Deng[2], P.K. Eagon[2], D.C. Whitcomb[2], D. Bimmler[1], R. Graf[1]

[1]Department of Visceral and Transplantation Surgery, University Hospital Zurich, Switzerland; [2]Division of Gastroenterology, Hepatology and Nutrition, University of Pittsburgh, PA, USA

Introduction: Alcoholics are more likely to develop both acute and chronic pancreatitis than non-alcoholics. In addition to alcohol, a second insult appears to be required to induce pancreatitis. The aim was to determine if an insult, i.e. LPS, exacerbates pancreatic injury in alcohol-fed animals.

Methods: Rats were fed a liquid diet (Lieber-DeCarli) containing either ethanol or maltose-dextrin in isocaloric amounts for 14 weeks and killed 24 h after endotoxin (LPS) injection (0.2, 0.8, 1.5 and 3 mg/kg bw). Pancreatic injury was assessed after tissue H&E staining by scoring parenchymal edema, acini necrosis, vacuolization, and inflammatory cell infiltration determined by Hemo Oxygenase (HO-1) IHC. Activities of caspase-3 (apoptosis executor), caspase-8 (receptor initiator) and caspase-9 (mitochondrial initiator) were investigated. Tissue necrosis was evaluated by measuring ATP deletion and the ratio of ADP/ATP.

Results: We show that chronic alcohol exposure alone inhibits apoptosis through the intrinsic pathway and the down-stream apoptosis executor caspase-3 when compared to controls. Pancreatic injury and inflammation increased after LPS injection in control and alcohol-fed rats in a dose-dependent fashion but with a significantly greater response in the alcohol-fed animals. Caspase activities were significantly lower in the alcoholic pancreas injected with LPS, while the histopathology and inflammation were more severe compared to control fed animals. Assessment of a putative indicator of necrosis, the ratio of ADP/ATP and ATP deletion indicated that alcohol exposure accelerate pancreatic necrosis in response to endotoxin.

Conclusions: This data suggest that damaged acinar cells cannot sufficiently be removed by apoptosis and enter necrotic cell death, with an exacerbation of pancreatic injury and necro-inflammation. We speculate that this mechanism may occur in acute alcoholic pancreatitis patients.

58

Lymphocytes Induce Increased Procollagen-1 mRNA Expression in Rat Pancreatic Stellate Cells

M. Grundsten[1], P. Hjelmström[2], B. Omazic[1], R. Segersvärd[1], J. Permert[1], J.A. Tsai[1]

[1]Division of Surgery and [2]Neurology, Karolinska Institutet at Karolinska University Hospital Huddinge, Stockholm, Sweden

Introduction: In chronic pancreatitis (CP) lymphocyte infiltrates in the pancreas are frequently seen, but it is unclear if these cells contribute to the pancreatic fibrosis. Pancreatic stellate cells (PSC) play a key role for the formation of pancreatic fibrosis. Our objective was to investigate interactions between PSCs and lymphocytes in an in vitro model using rat cells. We believe that these interactions are important for the pathogenesis of CP.

Methods: PSC and lymphocytes were isolated from the same rats. The two cell types were then co-cultured in a two-compartment well separated by a permeable membrane. In separate experiments, the co-culture was conducted by incubating both cell types in single-compartment wells. The latter experiments were also done using radiation-treated lymphocytes to eliminate DNA synthesis in these cells. DNA synthesis and procollagen-1 mRNA expression was measured with thymidine incorporation and realtime RT-PCR.

Results: Expression of procollagen-1 was increased 207% ($p = 0.04$, $n = 4$) after 24-hour co-culture with lymphocytes in the two-compartment setup. DNA synthesis in PSCs decreased 25% ($p = 0.002$, $n = 11$) in the two-compartment setup, but was unchanged after co-culture with lymphocytes or radiation-treated lymphocytes in the single-compartment setup.

Conclusions: In response to humoral lymphocytic stimulation the PSCs acted in two different ways. While the expression of procollagen-1 increased, DNA synthesis decreased. These results suggest that lymphocytes are important for formation of pancreatic fibrosis. Cell-cell interaction between PSCs and lymphocytes seems to counteract the humoral effect on DNA synthesis in PSCs.

59

Green Tea Catechin Prevents Ethanol-Induced Rat Pancreatic Stellate Cell Activation through Anti-Oxidative Effects

H. Asaumi, S. Watanabe, M. Taguchi, M. Tashiro, Y. Nagashio, Y. Nomiyama, T. Miyamoto, M. Otsuki

Department of Gastroenterology and Metabolism, University of Occupational and Environmental Health, Japan, School of Medicine, Kitakyushu, Japan

Introduction: Pancreatic stellate cells (PSCs) play a central role in the pancreatic fibrogenesis. Ethanol is a major cause of chronic pancreatitis, and known to activate PSCs through oxidative stress. Since inhibition of PSC activation might be a therapeutic strategy for prevention of pancreatic fibrosis, and since (–)-Epigallocatechin-3-gallate (EGCG), a major component of green tea extracts, is a potent antioxidant of polyphenols, we examined the mechanisms by which ethanol induces oxidative stress in PSCs and evaluated the effects of EGCG on ethanol-induced PSC activation.

Methods: PSCs were isolated from rat pancreas and cultured with ethanol (50 mM) in the absence or presence of EGCG (5, 25 μM). We assessed the effects of ethanol and EGCG on (i) oxidative stress in cell membrane by determining lipid peroxidation, (ii) oxidative stress in cytosol and mitochondria by measuring superoxide dismutase (SOD) activity and gene expression of Mn-SOD and Cu/Zn-SOD, (iii) α-SMA production by Western blotting, (iv) collagen secretion into the medium, (v) gene expression of TGF-β1, and (vi) phospholyration of p38 mitogen activated protein (MAP) kinase by Western blotting.

Results: Ethanol strongly increased lipid peroxidation in the cell membranes, and reduced SOD activity to 64.6% of the control at 24 h.

Ethanol also induced both Cu/Zn and Mn-SOD gene expressions. EGCG abolished ethanol-induced lipid peroxidation in the cell membrane, rescued SOD consumption to control levels and suppressed gene expression of both Cu/Zn and Mn-SOD. Ethanol increased α-SMA production, collagen secretion and TGF-β1 gene expression, and activated p38 MAP kinase. EGCG suppressed these ethanol-induced alterations in PSCs.

Conclusion: These results indicate that EGCG inhibits PSC activation through anti-oxidative effect. It is suggested that green tea and the polyphenols may prevent pancreatic fibrosis.

60

Determination of the Anti-Oxidant Status in the Liver and Pancreas of Neonatal and Adult Rats

A. Schneider, T. Hucl, A. Naeher, S. Tögel, P. Feick, M.V. Singer

Department of Medicine II, University Hospital of Heidelberg at Mannheim, Germany

Introduction: In hereditary pancreatitis, the attacks of acute pancreatitis usually begin in childhood. Several genetic mutations have been detected that cause the disease. However, additional individual factors most likely influence the disease expression and remain to be identified. Oxidative stress has been suggested to contribute to the development of pancreatitis. The aim was to characterize the anti-oxidant status in the liver and pancreas of neonatal and adult rats by determination of enzymatic activities of glutathione peroxidase (GPX) and catalase (CAT) and concentrations of reduced glutathione (GSH).

Methods: We determined GPX according to Lawrence and Burk (results in U/mg protein), CAT as described by Aebi (k/g protein), and GSH according to Tietze (nM/mg protein). Healthy male and female Sprague-Dawley rats were killed at postnatal days 1 and 15 and at adult age of 8–9 months.

Results: CAT activities were similar in the liver and pancreas of male and female rats and did not change significantly with increasing age. Liver GPX activities progressively increased from postnatal day 1 (51 ± 12; n = 5 male, n = 3 female) to adult age ($p < 0.05$). In adult rats, liver GPX activities were significantly different between male (277 ± 52; n = 6) and female ($p < 0.05$; 711 ± 134; n = 6) rats. Pancreatic GPX activities decreased from postnatal day 1 (46 ± 11; n = 5 males, n = 3 females) to day 15 ($p < 0.05$; 21 ± 8; n = 3 males, n = 6 females), and again increased to adult age (26 ± 10, n = 6 males vs. 33 ± 10, n = 6 females; p = ns). Liver GSH content progressively increased from postnatal day 1 (6.4 ± 2.1; n = 3 males, n = 3 females) to adult age ($p < 0.05$; 37.3 ± 10.8, n = 6 males; 31.3 ± 13.9, n = 6 females). In the pancreas, GSH content did not significantly change from day 1 (1.0 ± 0.2; n = 3 males, n = 3 females) to adult age 0.7 ± 0.1 (n = 6 males; n = 6 females).

Conclusions: The anti-oxidant systems in the liver and pancreas present different age- and gender-related patterns of development.

Experimental Pancreatic Cancer

61

Immunomodulatory Impact of Interferon-alpha in Combination with Chemoradiation of Pancreatic Adenocarcinoma (CapRI)

J. Schmidt, E.M. Patrut, J. Ma, H.-P. Knaebel, M.W. Büchler, A. Märten

Department of Surgery, University of Heidelberg, Germany

Introduction: Data from a phase II trial combining chemoradiotherapy with IFN-α (CapRI scheme) for adjuvant treatment of pancreatic carcinoma are very encouraging. Here, we have investigated the immunomodulatory effect of IFN-α in this regimen.

Methods: Eight human ductal pancreatic carcinoma cell lines were treated with the CapRI scheme (5-Fluorouracil, cisplatin, IFN-α and radiation). NK and T cells were preincubated with 1,000 U/ml IFN-α over 24 hours and tested in cytotoxicity assays against these cell lines and the mechanism of cell lysis was investigated. The induction of the immunoproteasome in tumor cells after IFN-α stimulation was analyzed by immunoblot and RT-PCR.

Results: Our results show an increase in cytotoxic activity of peripheral blood cells after IFN-α treatment from 12.5% to 34.3% ($p < 0.05$). This cytotoxicity was NK cell mediated as shown after depletion of T cells (T cells 4% lysis, NK cells 42.7% lysis) and was mediated as well by Fas-induced apoptosis as by perforin release. Pretreatment of tumor cells with 5-FU and combinations showed a significant increase in the susceptibility of tumor cells against NK cells (untreated tumor cells 34.3%, CapRI scheme 69.1%). Treatment of tumor cells with IFN-α induced a switch to the immunoproteasome and enhanced their vulnerability to T cells. This is the first description of this phenomenon in pancreatic carcinoma cells with implications for their immunogenicity.

Conclusions: IFN-α activates NK cells against pancreatic carcinoma cells and 5-FU treatment makes tumor cells more susceptible. Furthermore, IFN-α induces the immunoproteasome with impact on the immunogenicity of pancreatic carcinoma cells. These mechanisms may be responsible for the improved clinical outcome of CapRI.

62

Isolation and Characterization of Pancreatic Cancer Diabetogenic Factor: A 14 Aminoacids Peptide Corresponding to the N-Terminal Sequence of an S-100 Calcium Binding Protein

E. Greco[1], D. Basso[1], P. Fogar[2], P. Pucci[3], A. Flagiello[3], G. Baldo[2], S. Giunco[2], F. Navaglia[1], C.-F. Zambon[2], A. Falda[1], A. Valerio[4], S. Pedrazzoli[2], M. Plebani[1]

Departments of [1]Laboratory Medicine, [2]Medical and Surgical Sciences, [4]Clinical and Experimental Medicine, University of Padova; [3]CEINGE Advanced Biotechnologies and Department of Organic Chemistry and Biochemistry, University of Napoli, Italy

Introduction: Pancreatic cancer (PC)-associated diabetes is consequent to the action of a tumor peptide less than 10,000 Da. Our aim was to identify the PC-associated diabetogenic peptide.

Methods: Tumor homogenates from PC patients with (n = 15) or without (n = 8) diabetes, and normal pancreas homogenates (n = 6) were subjected to 16.5% SDS-PAGE. After Comassie staining a band of approximately 1500 Da was evidenced in tumor tissues only from diabetic PC. This band was cut and sequenced by automatic Adman degradation.

Results: The sequence obtained revealed a 14 a peptide of 1589.88 Da, corresponding to the N-terminal sequence of an S-100 calcium binding protein. This peptide was synthesized and its effects on glucose metabolism were tested in cultured C_2C_{12} my oblasts. These cells were cultured with different amounts (from 1 nmol/L to 2 mol/L) of the 14 a peptide. Glucose and lactate were measured in the supernatants after 24, 48 and 72 hours of incubation. In control my oblasts glucose concentration declined from 21.50 ± 0.48 mol/L (mean ± SE) to 6.3 ± 0.56, while lactate increased from 3.20 ± 0.08 mol/L to 34.50 ± 1.24 after 72 hours of incubation. 50 nmol/L 14 a peptide caused a significant reduction in glucose consumption and in lactate production after 72 hours of incubation with respect to control (Student's t test: $t = 3.87$, $p < 0.05$). At the same concentrations the 14 a peptide caused also my oblasts phenotypic alterations (accumulation of cells at the periphery of culture wells, lack of differentiation in myotubes and presence of polynucleated cells).

Conclusions: The N-terminal 14 aa peptide from an S-100 calcium binding protein is produced by PC causing diabetes mellitus; this peptide impairs glucose catabolism by myoblasts in vitro and this might determine hyperglycemia in vivo; its identification in patients' biological fluids might be helpful to diagnose PC when a recent onset diabetes mellitus occurs.

63

Midkine Promoter-Based Conditionally Replicative Adenovirus for Gene Therapy of Pancreatic Cancer

E. Toyoda[1,2], R. Doi[1], M. Wada[3], M. Tagawa[4], K. Hamada[5], K. Fujimoto[1]

[1]Department of Surgery and Surgical Basic Science, Kyoto University, Kyoto, [2]Shiga Medical Center for Adults, [3]Kobe City General Hospital, Kobe, [4]Division of Pathology, Chiba Cancer Center Research Institute, Chiba, [5]Department of Obstetrics and Gynecology, Ehime University, Ehime, Japan

Introduction: Midkine (MK) is a heparin-binding growth factor as a product of a retinoic acid-responsive gene. MK is highly expressed in many kinds of cancers; however, the expression of MK in human adult tissues is low and strictly limited. Therefore, MK promoter could be a potential candidate for suicide gene therapy. In this study, we investigated the efficacy of conditionally replicative adenovirus (Ad) in which expression of the essential E1 gene is driven by MK promoter (AdMK) on pancreatic cancer cells.

Methods: We examined the expression levels of MK in five human pancreatic cancer cell lines. The transcriptional activity of MK promoter fragment in cancer cells was measured with dual luciferase assay. The adenoviral transduction efficiency was examined by FACS analysis using Ad containing GFP gene. The selectivity of AdMK to cancer cells was assessed by Western blot analyses with anti-Ad E1A antibodies. The cytotoxicity of AdMK in vitro was determined by comparing the cell count of MK positive cells with negative cells after AdMK infection.

Results: All of the cell lines except MIAPaCa-2 expressed MK gene at varying degrees. The transcriptional activity was almost parallel to the expression level of MK except CFPAC-1. Ad transduction efficiency of four cell lines was moderate or high except AsPc-1, whereas it was extremely low in AsPc-1. E1A expression in MK-positive cells was higher than that of low MK-expressing cells. Viral replication was depended on an MOI of infected cells. AdMKp showed much effective cell-killing activity in MIAPaCa-2 MK-negative cells, although it was hardly found in AsPc-1 which highly expressed MK.

Conclusions: The results suggest that the use of oncolytic adenoviruses using MK promoter may be a good tool for the therapy of human pancreatic cancer. Moreover, we conclude that Ad transduction efficiency is very important for Ad-mediated gene therapy.

64

Morphological Patterns of Human Pancreatic Cancer Xenografts are Associated with Molecular Markers of Trans- and De-Differentiation

D. Neureiter[1], S. Zopf[2], A. Dimmler[1], S. Stintzing[2], E.G. Hahn[2], T. Kirchner[1], C. Herold[2], M. Ocker[2]

[1]Department of Pathology, [2]Department of Medicine I, Friedrich-Alexander-University Erlangen-Nürnberg, Germany

Aims: New concepts of tumorigenesis favor an unregulated process recapitulating different stages of embryogenic development with dysregulation of transition states. The aim of our study was to investigate the possibility of differentiation pathways of human pancreatic cancer cell lines in vivo.

Material and Methods: Different human pancreatic cancer cell lines (YAPC, DAN-G, CAPAN-1, PANC-1 and MIA PaCa-2) were implanted subcutaneously (3×10^6 cells) for 28 days in nude mice. Xenotransplants were characterized with histochemistry (HE, PAS), immunohistochemistry (cytokeratin (CK)7, CK8, CK18, CK19, CK20, vimentin, chromogranin A, α1-antichymotrypsin, β-catenin, laminin-1, pancreatic and duodenal homeobox gene 1 (pdx-1), sonic hedgehog protein (shh), patched (ptc)), Western blotting and real-time-PCR (CK7, CK8, CK20, chromogranin A, pdx-1, shh, ptc).

Results: Depending on three major morphologic phenotypes of tumor cell xenotransplants (ductal (YAPC), ductal/solid (DAN-G, CAPAN-1), solid (PANC-1, MIA PaCa-2)), a decrease of CK7/CK19 was found, accompanied by an increase of CK8/18 and vimentin. Predominantly the CK7 positive ductal phenotype (YAPC and DAN-G) was associated with pdx-1 expression, whereas the CK8 positive solid phenotype was associated with shh/ptc expression on protein and mRNA level. Additionally, CK-20 expression was mainly linked to the ductal phenotype, co-localized with nuclear β-catenin. The endocrine-exocrine trans-differentiation, as assessed by chromogranin A and α1-antichymotrypsin, was on a constant low to moderate level in all xenotransplants. Finally, an intensive epithelial-mesenchymal interaction was observed by overexpression of laminin-1 at the invasion front.

Conclusion: The observed patterns of morphology and molecular markers of transition states seem to indicate that specific morphology is linked to specific pathways of trans-differentiation as well as of embryonic pancreatic development.

65

siRNA-Based Approaches to Pancreatic Cancer

M. Ocker[1], D. Neureiter[2], M. Lüders[1], S. Zopf[1], M. Ganslmayer[1], E.G. Hahn[1], C. Herold[1]

[1]Department of Medicine 1 and [2]Department of Pathology, Friedrich-Alexander-University Erlangen-Nürnberg, Germany

Introduction: Pancreatic cancer remains a devastating diagnosis with only limited therapeutic options. Specific inhibition of the expression of target genes has become possible using small interfering (si)RNAs. We therefore investigated how far siRNA specific for bcl-2 may serve as a therapeutic option for pancreatic cancer in vitro and in vivo and if this treatment sensitizes tumor cells to treatment with gemcitabine.

Methods: siRNAs targeting two different regions in the bcl-2 gene were transfected to YAP C pancreatic carcinoma cells and human foreskin fibroblasts. Transfection efficacy was determined using FITC-labeled siRNAs and fluorescence microscopy. Cell survival and apoptosis were quantified at 24 to 120 h. YAP C-xenografts in male nude-mice were treated intraperitoneally with siRNAs daily for 24 days. siRNA pharmacokinetics in vivo were assessed using radioactively labeled siRNAs. Total protein and RNA were extracted for Western Blot analysis and quantitative PCR. Cells were treated with gemcitabine in different concentrations for 24 to 120 h alone or 72 h after transfection of 10 nM bcl-2-specific siRNA. The above described parameters were assessed.

Results: bcl-2-specific siRNAs specifically inhibited the expression of the target gene in vitro and in vivo. Synergistic effects of silencing bcl-2 and treatment with gemcitabine were observed in YAP C leading to increased apoptosis at otherwise ineffective concentrations of the chemotherapeutic agent. Anti-proliferative and pro-apoptotic effects were observed in tumor cells but not in fibroblasts or non-malignant tissues in vivo. siRNA was quickly distributed to all organs and excreted via kidney and liver.

Conclusion: bcl-2-specific siRNA is a promising adjunctive treatment for pancreatic carcinoma.

Supported by grants for the German Cancer Aid, ELAN-Fonds at the University Erlangen-Nürnberg and the FUTUR-Program of the State of Bavaria.

66

Hypoxia Inducible Factor-1alpha (HIF-1α) in Pancreatic Cancer Cells is Involved in the Cell's Tumorigenicity in Nude Mice and the Cell's Impact on the Host's Energy Homeostasis

F. Wang[1], S.S. Li[2], R. Segersvärd[1], L. Strömmer[1], K.G. Sundqvist[2], J. Holgersson[2], J. Permert[1]

Departments of [1]Surgery and [2]Clinical Immunology, Karolinska Institute, Huddinge, Sweden

Introduction: Hypoxia inducible factor 1alpha (HIF-1α) is expressed in different malignant tumors including pancreatic carcinoma. We have demonstrated that HIF-1α in pancreatic cancer cells mediates trophic effects of insulin on the cancer cells. In the present study, we investigated whether HIF-1α in MiaPaCa2 human pancreatic cancer cells was involved in tumor-host interaction after the cells were transplanted orthotopically in nude mice.

Methods: We conducted the present study using three MiaPaCa2 cell types, namely (i) si_{HIF}-MiaPaCa2, which were transduced by lentiviruses to produce short interfering RNA inhibiting HIF-1α expression, (ii) cv-MiaPaCa2, which were transduced by control lentiviruses having no effects on gene expression, and (iii) wt-MiaPaCa2 (wild type). These cells were transplanted, respectively, in the pancreas of nude mice (one-million cells per pancreas). After transplantation, mice were kept for 16 weeks before being sacrificed to check the cancer cells' tumorigenicity. Energy homeostasis was characterized in these cancer-cell recipients. The metabolic data were compared to control values derived from a group of intact nude mice.

Results: The two HIF-1α-expressing cell lines, i.e. wt- and cv-MiaPaCa2, formed pancreatic tumors in 6/8 and 7/8 of their hosts, respectively (collective tumorigenicity: 13/16, 81%). In contrast, si_{HIF}MiaPaCa2 cell's tumorigenicity was significantly less, as pancreatic tumors were seen in three of nine mice transplanted with the cells (33%, $p < 0.05$). By the end of the 16-week study, body weight gain in mice transplanted with wt- and cv-MiaPaCa2 cells (6.4 ± 0.5 g, n = 16) was significantly less than that in control mice (9.1 ± 0.7 g, n = 8, $p < 0.05$). In contrast, body weight gain in mice transplanted with si_{HIF}-MiaPaCa2 cells (7.3 ± 0.7 g, n = 9) was not significantly different from the control value. Finally, mice in the four groups showed similar results in intra-peritoneal glucose tolerance test.

Conclusion: HIF-1α is involved in pancreatic cancer cell's survival and the cell's impact on host energy homeostasis.

67

Expression Profile of sst2 Somatostatin Receptor in Intraductal Papillary and Mucinous Tumors of the Pancreas: A New Tumor Suppressor Gene?

F. Marrache[1,2], A. Couvelard[3], P. Rochaix[4], P. Hammel[2], P. Cordelier[1], C. Susini[1], A. Sauvanet[5], P. Lévy[2], P. Ruszniewski[2], L. Buscail[1]

[1]Unité Inserm U 531, Institut Louis Bugnard, CHU Rangueil, Toulouse, [2]Service de Gastroentérologie, Hôpital Beaujon, Clichy, [3]Service d'Anatomie et Cytologie Pathologiques, Hôpital Beaujon, Clichy, [4]Service d'Anatomie et Cytologie Pathologiques, Institut Claudius Regaud, Toulouse, [5]Service de chirurgie digestive, Hôpital Beaujon, Clichy, France

Introduction: Somatostatin receptor sst2 is involved in the negative control of cell proliferation. Its expression is lost in 90% of pancreatic adenocarcinoma and it has been shown to have an anti-tumoral effect when re-expressed in pancreatic cancer models. All these observations suggested a role of sst2 in pancreatic carcinogenesis. The aim of this work was to clarify this role by study sst2 expression profile using intraductal papillary and mucinous tumors of the pancreas (IPMT) as model of pancreatic carcinogenesis.

Material and Methods: Immunohistochemistry for sst2 was performed on 54 IPMT lesions from 44 surgical specimens. IPMT lesions were classified as benign (n = 11), borderline (n = 9), malignant non invasive (n = 23) and malignant invasive (n = 11). Controls were non tumoral pancreas (n = 5) and non IPMT pancreatic adenocarcinoma (n = 4).

Results: Sst2 expression increased with malignancy in IPMT (see table). Conversely its expression was faint in a single case of non IPMT pancreatic carcinoma.

Moreover, expression of sst2 was found in foci of acinar regression and in the epithelium of pancreatic hyperplastic ducts of chronic pancreatitis lesions surrounding IPMT. Among non IPMT pancreatic adenocarcinoma, a single specimen faintly expressed sst2 in 10% of cells. In non tumoral pancreas without chronic pancreatitis, sst2 expression was found in islet cells, and in few pancreatic ducts.

IPMT grade	Positive specimens	Percentage of positive cells
Benign	0/11	0
Borderline	2/9 (22.2%)	30
Malignant non-invasive	12/23 (52.1%)	33.6 ± 10
Malignant invasive	5/11 (45.5%)	35.5 ± 19

Conclusion: Expression of sst2 is found in conditions of increased cellular proliferation (malignant forms of IPMT and chronic pancreatitis lesions), whereas it is faintly expressed in non IPMT pancreatic adenocarcinoma. These results show that sst2 expression is induced late during pancreatic carcinogenesis suggesting it acts as a sensor for controlling aberrant pancreatic proliferating tissues.

68

Stellate Cells Contribute to Create a Tumor-Favourable Environment in Pancreatic Cancer

I. Esposito[1], R. Penzel[1], F. Bergmann[1], N. Giese[2], J. Kleeff[2], H. Friess[2], P. Schirmacher[1]

[1]Institute of Pathology, [2]Department of General Surgery, University of Heidelberg, Heidelberg, Germany

Introduction: Tenascin C (TNC) is an extracellular matrix protein involved in tumor progression, in part through its binding to cell surface receptors, such as annexin II. The aim of this study was to analyze the expression and the regulation of TNC in pancreatic ductal adenocarcinoma (PDAC), which is characterized by a dense desmoplastic stroma populated by fibroblast-like cells (stellate cells).

Methods: TNC and annexin II mRNA expression levels in human pancreatic tissues, cancer cell lines and pancreatic stellate cells were analyzed by cDNA array and quantitative RT-PCR. Immunohistochemistry was used to localize and quantify the expression of TNC and annexin II in PDAC and its precursor lesions (PanIN). TNC large splice variants were detected by RT-PCR and quantified in serum and culture supernatants by ELISA.

Results: TNC and annexin II mRNA levels were significantly higher in pancreatic cancer tissues than in the normal pancreas (4- and 2-fold increase, respectively). TNC mRNA was demonstrated in pancreatic stellate cells, where it could be induced by TNFα and to a lesser extent by TGFβ-1 and cancer cell supernatants. Stromal TNC expression was detected with increased frequency from low-grade PanIN lesions to PDAC and a parallel redistribution of annexin II from the cytoplasm to the cell membrane was observed. Large TNC transcripts were shown in PDAC but not in the normal pancreas, however TNC serum levels did not significantly differ between patients with PDAC and normal controls.

Conclusions: Paracrine epithelial-stromal interactions lead to an increasing accumulation of TNC in the pancreatic stroma, which parallels annexin II expression on the cell surface and accompanies pancreatic cancer progression from pre-invasive PanIN lesions to invasive PDAC.

69

Characterisation of in vivo Model Systems of Human Pancreatic Cancer

H. Petznek[1], A. Url[2], J. Hlavaty[1], H. Holzmüller[3], G. Jandl[1], B. Salmons[3], W.H. Günzburg[1], M. Renner[3]

[1]Research Institute of Virology and Biomedicine, [2]Institute of Pathology and Forensic Veterinary Medicine, Department of Pathobiology, Veterinary University of Medicine, Vienna, [3]Austrianova Biotechnology GmbH, Vienna, Austria

Introduction: Pancreatic cancer represents a severe disease with an extremely poor prognosis. In order to evaluate new treatment strategies as gene therapy to combat this disease, defined animal models are needed. Here, we evaluate the use of six human pancreatic cancer cell lines in subcutaneous (s.c.) and intraperitoneal (i.p.; orthotopically growing cells) mouse models. In addition, sensitivity towards chemotherapeutic drugs ifosfamide (IFO), 5-fluorouracil (5-FU), and 5-fluorocytosine (5-FC) was examined in parental cells and in retrovirally transduced cells expressing cytochrome 2B1 (CYP 2B1) and cytosine deaminase (CD) genes, respectively.

Methods: PaCa-44, Panc-1, MiaPaca-2, Hs-766T, Capan-2 and BxPc-3 cells were either injected s.c. into the left flank of C.B.-17/IcrHsd-*Prkdc^{scid}Lyst^{bg}* mice or as already established tumours orthotopically implantated in close proximity to the pancreas. Tumour take and growth rate of the s.c. tumours were determined for both models and detailed pathohistological and immunohistochemical investigations performed. An XTT assay was used to evaluate the effect of the CYP2B1 and CD gene transfer on the sensitivity of transduced cells towards IFO, 5-FU, and 5-FC.

Results: Tumour uptake was 83.4 to 100% in the s.c. model and 60 to 100% in the i.p. model, except for HS766T cells, which did not grow i.p.. Pathohistological analyses of the i.p. models showed an infiltrative growth of the tumours into the pancreas albeit lacking large necrotic areas which have been seen, however, in the s.c. model. All of the tumours are positive for Muc 1 staining indicating their ductal origin or their dedifferentiation into ductal cells. Expression of suicide genes (CYP2B1, CD) leads to decreased viability in the presence of low concentrations of IFO or 5-FC.

Conclusions: The orthotopic models described here are a valuable tool for defined preclinical studies of new therapeutic agents. Suicide gene therapy in these models may represent a promising approach in the treatment of pancreatic cancer.

70

Smad3/4 and Sp1 mediate the TGFβ-Induced Expression of Smad7 in Pancreatic Carcinoma Cells

K. Jungert, A. Buck, A. Harth, A. Schatz, G. Adler, T.M. Gress, V. Ellenrieder

Department of Internal Medicine I, University of Ulm, Germany

Introduction: In healthy epithelial cells, TGFβ acts as a tumor suppressor by inducing a cell cycle arrest, whereas in late tumor stages the anti-proliferatve action is lost. On cellular level, TGFβ signalling is mediated by phosphorylation of Smad2 and Smad3 through activated TGFβ receptors. Phosphorylated Smad2/3 form a complex with Smad4. This complex translocates into the nucleus and, together with specific transcription factors, controls the expression of TGFβ target genes. The transcription factor Sp1 is an important cofactor for Smad-mediated regulation of promoters and, besides, has a role in the expression of tumor progressor genes. In order to identify tumor-associated target genes in Panc1 cells, whose regulation is mediated by both TGFβ and Sp1, we performed expression profiling.

Methods: The expression of TGFβ target genes in Panc1 cells was analysed by expression profiling analysis and quantitative RT-PCR. Panc1 cells were stimulated with TGFβ and compared to cells that were coincubated with Mithramycin, an agent that inhibits the binding of Sp1 to its DNA consensus sequences. Protein detection was performed by western blot and immunofluorescence. Protein-protein interaction was examined in immunoprecipitation experiments. Promoter studies were performed by reporter- and DNA pulldown assays.

Results: Various genes, where the coincubation of mithramycin had an opposing effect on TGFβ mediated regulation, were identified by expression profiling. One of them was the inhibitory Smad7, whose increased expression in pancreatic carcinoma cells is associated with the loss of TGFβ mediated growth inhibition. Promoter studies confirmed, that Sp1 is required for full Smad3/4 mediated activation of the Smad7 promoter. Furthermore, the results of immunoprecipitation and DNA pulldown experiments suggest a mechanism, in which Smad3/4-Sp1 interaction leads to increased binding of Sp1 to the Smad7 promoter.

Conclusion: The transcription factor Sp1 plays a central role in the Smad3/4 mediated expression of Smad7 in pancreatic carcinoma cells.

71

Pancreatic Cancer Gene Therapy Using rH1-yCD Autonomous Parvovirus with Carcinoembryonic Antigen/P4 Chimeric Promoter

S. Réjiba, G. Balboni, M. Aprahamian, A. Hajri

INSERM U701, IRCAD, Strasbourg, France

Background: Successful gene therapy depends on the development of safe and efficient vectors for gene expression targeting.

We investigated the use of a rH1CEA-yCD recombinant parvoviral vector, bearing the yeast cytosine deaminase (yCD) suicide gene. The parvoviral P4 promoter was modified by the addition of a 319 bp carcinoembryonic antigen (CEA) tissue-specific promoter sequence, to improve the oncotropic and oncolytic intrinsic properties of the H-1 parvovirus.

Material and Methods: To this end, we explored in vitro, the ability of this rH1CEA-yCD virus to infect CEA-producing cell lines (BxPc3) and CEA-nonproducing cell lines (HA-HPC and HeLa). For in vivo experiments, we evaluated this new recombinant parvovirus on tumor growth upon subcutaneous/peritoneal pancreatic carcinomatosis models in nude mice.

Results: Our data indicate that rH1CEA-yCD infect efficiently the tumor cell lines in the same manner as its parental rH1-yCD. RT-PCR and western blot analyses showed a down-regulation of the expression of both the NS1 (viral gene) and the yCD (suicide gene) brought by rH1CEA-yCD in HA-HPC and HeLa cell lines, when compared with rH1-yCD. With regard to its cytotoxic effect, rH1CEA-yCD/5-FC treatment was incapable to induce cell death in those cell lines, but was as efficient as rH1-yCD to kill BxPc3 cell line. In vivo, infection with rH1CEA-yCD led to significant retardation of BxPc3 tumor growth both in subcutaneous and intraperitoneal disseminated pancreatic models. The survival rate of animals bearing CEA-producing cell lines (BxPc3) was prolonged ($p < 0.001$). However, there was no effect on HA-HPC tumor models.

Conclusion: In summary, we have developed a new targeted recombinant parvovirus where the parvoviral oncolytic effect and the suicide gene expression are tightly restricted to tumor cells with CEA tumor marker promoter signaling.

72

Chemosensitivity of Human Pancreatic Cancer Cell Lines Expressing Galα1,3Gal Xenoantigen

M. Ouaïssi[1,2], M.O. Sadoulet[1], F. Silvy[1], M. Aubert[3], C. Franceschi[1], B. Sastre[2], D. Lombardo[1], J.P. Bernard[1], E. Mas[1]

[1]Inserm U559, Faculté de Médecine-Timone, [2] Service de Chirurgie Digestive, Hôpital Ste Marguerite, Marseille, France; [3]Imperial College Faculty of Medicine, Hammersmith Hospital, London, UK

Background: Many modifications in glycosylation of cell surface glycoconjugates have been described in pancreatic adenocarcinoma. These modifications were often correlated with aggressiveness, invasion, metastasis and tumor progression of pancreatic tumoral cells and could be associated with resistance to drugs used in chemotherapy. We have previously shown that Galα1,3Gal carbohydrate structure (αGal epitope) expression, a xenoantigen which participates in the hyperacute rejection of xenograft, by human pancreatic tumoral cells decreases the tumorigenic behavior of these cells. The aim of this study was to determine whether the expression of αGal epitope can modify the susceptibility of human pancreatic cancer cells to chemotherapeutic drugs.

Methods: The expression of αGal epitopes in the human pancreatic cancer cell lines BxPC-3 and Panc-1 was obtained by selecting stable cell clones transfected with murine α1,3galactosyltransferase gene. In vitro cell growth assays recorded by [^{3}H]-thymidine incorporation were performed in presence of cisplatin, gemcitabin or 5-FU. Nude mice were implanted subcutaneously with Panc-1 cells expressing the αGal epitope or with control cells to generate tumors and were treated with cisplatin.

Results: Compared to control cells, the in vitro treatment of Panc-1 cells expressing αGal epitopes with cisplatin result to a 50% inhibition of cell proliferation at 30 min followed by the cell death. This cell death seems to be induced by necrotic rather than apoptotic pathways. In vivo studies conducted in nude mice after xenograft transplantation of Panc-1 cells expressing αGal epitopes and cisplatin treatment showed a delay in the tumoral development compared to control xenografts.

Conclusions: The expression of the αGal xenoantigen could induce an increased susceptibility of human pancreatic cancer cells to cisplatine treatment. The de novo expression of the αGal epitope by tumoral cells represents a good challenge in the development of new therapeutic strategy in gene immunotherapy combined with chemotherapy of pancreatic cancer.

73

Occult Tumor Cells in Lymph Nodes as a Predictor for Tumor Relapse in Pancreatic Cancer

P. Scheunemann[1], N.H. Stoecklein[1], A. Rehders[1], M. Bidde[2], P.E. Verde[3], J. Schulte am Esch[1], S. Metz[2], M. Peiper[1], C. Eisenberger[1], W.T. Knoefel[1], S.B. Hosch[1]

[1]Klinik für Allgemein- und Visceralchirurgie, Universitätsklinikum Düsseldorf, Germany, [2]Klinik für Allgemein-, Visceral- und Thoraxchirurgie, Universitätsklinikum Hamburg, Germany, [3]Koordinationszentrum für klinische Studien, Universitätsklinikum Düsseldorf, Germany

Background: Occurrence of tumor relapse is frequent in patients with pancreatic cancer despite the absence of residual tumor detectable at primary surgery. Therefore it has to be assumed that current tumor staging procedures fail to identify minimal amounts of tumor cells disseminated to secondary organs, which might be precursors of subsequent metastatic relapse. The aim of the study was to assess the frequency and prognostic impact of minimal tumor cell spread in lymph nodes classified as 'tumor free' in routine histopathologic evaluation.

Methods: We examined in total 209 lymph nodes judged as 'tumor-free' by routine histopathology from 90 patients with pancreatic cancer without overt metastases (M0) who had undergone intentional curative tumor resection. Isolated tumor cells were detected by immunohistochemistry with the monoclonal antiepithelial antibody Ber-EP4.

Results: Sixty-six (31.6%) of the 209 'tumor-free' lymph nodes obtained from 49 (54.4%) of these 90 patients displayed Ber-EP4+ cells. No correlation was found between immunohistochemical detection of Ber-EP4+ cells in 'tumor-free' lymph nodes and histopathological parameters, such as primary tumor stage (pT), lymph node stage (pN), histological tumor type or tumor grading (G).

Postoperative Kaplan-Meier survival analyses revealed that patients with Ber-EP4+ cells in 'tumor-free' lymph nodes had both a significantly reduced relapse-free survival ($p = 0.0006$) and overall survival ($p = 0.0003$). Interestingly, only metastatic relapse-free survival was significantly reduced in patients with Ber-EP4+ cells in lymph nodes ($p = 0.0047$) whereas local recurrence-free survival was not ($p = 0.43$). Furthermore, multivariate Cox regression analysis confirmed the presence of Ber-EP4+ cells in 'tumor-free' lymph nodes as an independent prognostic factor for a significantly reduced relapse-free survival and overall survival ($p = 0.001$ and $p < 0.0001$, respectively).

Conclusion: The frequent occurrence and prognostic impact of early disseminated tumor cells in lymph nodes of patients with operable pancreatic cancer support the need for a refined staging system of excised lymph nodes, which should include immunohistochemical examination.

74

Chemoresistance of Pancreatic Tumors – A Proteome Analysis

R. Faissner[1], A. Funk[1], S. Wandschneider[2], M. Schnölzer[2], M. Löhr[1]

[1]Department of Medicine II, Mannheim Medical Faculty, University of Heidelberg, Germany, [2]Central Protein Analysis, DKFZ, Heidelberg, Germany

Background: Tumors of the pancreas are characterized by a high potency to develop chemoresistance towards cytostatic drugs, which is the main cause of ineffective treatment. The biological mechanisms of this resistance are still unknown. We used a proteomic approach to analyse protein regulation of pancreatic cell lines treated with cytostatic drugs.

Methods: Three human pancreatic cancer cell lines (PANC-1, Paca44, CAPAN-1) were treated with 5-FU, gemcitabine and mafosfamide for 24 hours. A 5-FU-resistant CAPAN-1 cell line was developed through exposure to increasing concentrations of 5-FU. High-resolution 2D-gels were produced (IEF, SDS-PAGE) and the resulting gels were stained and digitalized. Image analysis was performed (PDQuest) and differentially regulated proteins were excised from the gel, digested, and submitted to mass spectrometry (MALDI-TOF-MS). Proteins were identified by Peptide Mass Fingerprint (PMF).

Results: We identified more than 80 cell line protein spots to date. Image analysis showed that more than 10 protein spots are differentially regulated – one of them identified as annexin IV. Work is ongoing to identify all differentially expressed proteins.

Conclusions: The proteomic approach is a solid and reproducible method for identifying differentially regulated proteins. Identification of chemoresistance-related proteins will further our understanding of the biological mechanism of chemoresistance and may lead to novel cyctostatic drugs.

75

The Thrombin Receptor PAR-1 Plays an Important Role in Pancreatic Cancer Cell Invasiveness in vitro

C. Rudroff[1], U. Schaefer[2], S. Seibold[3], M.M. Heiss[1]

[1]Department of Visceral, Vascular and Transplant Surgery, University of Witten-Herdecke, Krankenhaus Köln-Merheim, Germany, [2]Department of Experimental Surgery, University of Cologne, Germany, [3]Department of Medicine, University of Würzburg, Germany

Background: Thrombosis and activation of coagulation are frequently observed in cancer patients. This phenomenon is reflected in the excess production of thrombin, which is thought to play an important role the progression of different solid tumors. Cellular effects of thrombin are mediated by the thrombin receptor PAR-1, a member of the G-protein coupled receptor family. Aim of this study was to investigate the role of PAR-1 on pancreatic cancer cell invasion.

Material and Methods: The human pancreatic cancer cell line MIA PaCa-2, which expresses high levels of PAR-1, was transfected with an antisense construct against PAR-1. The expression level of PAR-1 after transfection was determined by RT-PCR and Western blot analysis. For invasion assays the respective transfected, control transfected (sense and mock) and untransfected cells were stimulated with thrombin (1.0 U/ml) and subjected to a standardized matrigel invasion assay. After 24 hours the number of invasive cells were counted.

Results: Antisense transfection resulted in 80% down regulation of PAR-1 expression compared to parental MIA PaCa-2. In the Matrigel invasion assay the number of invasive cells was significantly reduced for the antisense transfected cells. The control transfected cells showed no change of invasiveness compared to untransfected MIA PaCa-2.

Conclusion: The expression of the thrombin receptor PAR-1 was succesfully reduced in pancreatic cancer cells by antisense transfection. Down regulation of the thrombin receptor lead to significantly reduced invasiveness in vitro. These results emphasize the crucial role of PAR-1 in pancreatic cancer progression in vitro. In vivo assays to confirm the impact of PAR-1 expression on pancreatic cancer cell invasiveness are prospected.

76

The Proteomic Identification of Autoantibodies Prevalent in Pancreatic Cancer Serum

S. Shore, C.C.M. Thompson, J.P. Neoptolemos, P. Ghaneh, E. Costello

Division of Surgery and Oncology, University of Liverpool, Liverpool, UK

Introduction: Pancreatic cancer remains one of the most deadly cancers in the western world, due in part to its asymptomatic nature and difficulty in diagnosis, resulting in the treatment of often advanced disease. A simple blood test would be ideal for high risk patients or patients with vague symptoms. Autoantibodies to pancreatic cancer have already been identified in serum but usually at low proportions. Using proteomic techniques we have screened cancer serum for unknown autoantibodies.

Methods: Protein cellular extracts from five pancreatic ductal adenocarcinoma (PDAC) samples (>70% tumour) were separated using 2-dimensional electrophoresis. Ten gels were prepared from each tumour sample. Proteins were transferred onto PVDF membranes and probed with either cancer serum, benign serum or secondary only horseradish peroxidase antibody. Detection was by electro-chemiluminesence. Spot profiles were compared and spots predominantly present in cancer sera-probed blots were identified. These spots identify possible immunogenic proteins in PDAC. For spot identification, immunoblot profiles were aligned with Coomassie blue stained gels. Spots of interest were extracted and subjected to mass spectrometric analysis.

Results: In total 13 cancer and 12 benign sera were blotted against 5 tumours. Eleven spots were found to be more prevalent in blots probed with cancer sera than normal sera. These spots were present in between 7/13 to 9/13 of the cancer sera (54–69%), but only present in 0/12 to 3/12 of benign sera (0–25%). Protein putatively identified as autoantibody targets are being validated against a larger number of sera.

Conclusions: Eleven proteins appear to induce an auto-immune response more prevalent in cancer than normal serum. Their reciprocal autoantibodies could be used to detect pancreatic cancer at an earlier stage.

Funding received from the Royal College of Surgeons of England, and the Royal Liverpool and Broadgreen University Hospital.

77

Opioid Growth Factor (OGF) Enhances the Inhibitory Effect of Gemcitabine on the Growth of Pancreatic Adenocarcinoma

J.P. Smith[1], J.R. Jaglowski[2], M.F. Verderame[1], A.E. Leure-duPree[2], P.J. McLaughlin[2], I.S. Zagon[2]

Departments of [1]Medicine and [2]Neural and Behavioral Sciences, The Pennsylvania State University College of Medicine, Hershey, PA, USA

Introduction: Gemcitabine is the standard of care for advanced pancreatic neoplasia; however, gemcitabine has limited survival benefits. Recently, OGF ([Met^5]-enkephalin) has been shown to inhibit pancreatic cancer growth in animals and human subjects through the OGF receptor. The present study was designed to examine whether the combination of gemcitabine and OGF is more effective than either agent alone in pancreatic cancer.

Methods: In vitro, human pancreatic cancer cells (MIA PaCa-2 and Panc-1) were exposed to 10^{-6} M OGF or 10^{-8} M gemcitabine, or both in combination; cells were seeded for 24 hr prior to daily treatments. Cell growth was recorded at 24, 48, 72, and 96 hr in culture using the MTS proliferation assay. In vivo, MIA PaCa-2 tumor cells were inoculated subcutaneously into nude mice, and mice were treated daily with OGF (10 mg/kg) or gemcitabine (120 mg/kg) every 3rd day, or a combination of OGF and gemcitabine; controls received sterile saline daily. Animal weights and tumor volumes were measured, and on day 45, the mice were sacrificed and tumors dissected and weighed.

Results: In vitro, the combination of OGF and gemcitabine markedly inhibited growth of both pancreatic cancer cell lines compared to control-treated cells or single agents. Tumor incidence and latency times to tumor appearance, of mice receiving combined therapy, were significantly decreased from the control, OGF, and gemcitabine groups. On day 10, tumor incidence was the following: 80%, saline control mice, 75% gemcitabine, 60% OGF, and 0% combination. Compared to controls, final tumor weights were decreased by 36%, 56%, and 85%, respectively for the OGF, gemcitabine, and combination groups.

Conclusions: These data provide preclinical evidence that combined chemotherapy (gemcitabine) and biotherapy (OGF) has an enhanced therapeutic benefit for treatment of human pancreatic cancer.

Supported by Philip Morris Inc. and a Tobacco Settlement Grant.

78

A New Combined Therapy of an Oncolytic Replication-Competent HSV-1 Vector Using Survivin Promoter and Radiation for Pancreatic Cancer

K. Kami[1], R. Doi[1], S.-I. Miyatake[2], M. Imamura[1]

[1]Department of Surgery and Surgical Basic Science, Kyoto University, [2]Department of Neurosurgery, Osaka Medical College, Japan

Introduction: We constructed an oncolytic HSV-1 vector (d120.survE) using survivin promoter which replicates selectively in survivin expressing cells. Survivin expresses in cancer cells specifically, and is considered to be a radio-resistant factor for pancreatic cancer cells. We assessed the ability of d120.survE and/or radiation to inhibit the growth of pancreatic cancer cells.

Methods: (1) Survivin promoter activity was measured using luciferase assay and survivin mRNA expression was quantified using TaqMAN PCR in cells with and without radiation treatment. (2) A transgene (TK promoter-LacZ-survivin promoter-ICP4) was cloned into tk gene of the mutant HSV-1 d120 which lacks ICP4 gene, to generate d120.suvE. (3) In vitro studies; ICP4 and LacZ expression were examined by RT-PCR and X-gal staining. The ability of d120.survE to replicate and the cytotoxic effect of d120.survE in cells treated with and without radiation were examined. (4) In vivo studies; Nude mice harboring AsPC-1 tumors subcutaneously received once on day1 intraneoplasmic injection of d120.survE after treatment with radiation once on day0 (0 Gy or 5 Gy). The tumor sizes were measured every 5 days.

Results: (1) Survivin promoter activity was associated with survivin mRNA expression. Survivin expression was correlated with radio-sensitivity, and was increased after radiation in pancreatic cancer cell lines. (3) ICP4 and LacZ were expressed in the cells infected with d120.survE. The ability of d120.survE to replicate and the cytotoxic effect of d120.survE were correlated with survivin promoter activity of the host cells, and they were augmented after radiation treatment. (4) Subcutaneous tumors treated with d120.survE were significantly smaller than control tumors by day70 post-infection. Tumors treated with radiation and vector were significantly smaller than tumors treated with vector alone. ICP4 and LacZ expression were observed in the tumors treated with the vector.

Conclusion: A combined therapy of d120.survE and radiation may be a useful treatment of pancreatic cancer.

79

Aurora Kinase A is Involved in Tumor Growth and Taxane Chemosensitivity in Human Pancreatic Cancer

M. Sunamura[1], T. Hata[2], T. Furukawa[2], S. Egawa[1], F. Motoi[1], N. Ohmura[1], T. Marumoto[3], H. Saya[3], A. Horii[2]

Departments of [1]Gastroenterological Surgery and [2]Molecular Pathology, Tohoku University School of Medicine, Sendai, Japan, [3]Department of Tumor Genetics and Biology, Graduate School of Medical Sciences, Kumamoto University, Kumamoto, Japan

Background: Pancreatic cancer involves very complicated molecular changes. Our previous comparative genomic hybridization (CGH) analysis of the pancreatic cancer genome revealed intricate genomic alterations in multiple chromosome arms, including losses of 1p, 3p, 4q, 6q, 8p, 9p, 12q, 17p, 18q, and 21q and gains of 8q and 20q. The increase in copy number of 20q13 is especially prominent in pancreatic cancer. Amplification of 20q13 is also found in several other types of human cancer, suggesting the existence of an important oncogene(s) that plays a crucial role in a variety of human cancers in this area. AURKA was identified as one of the candidate oncogenes from the amplicon on 20q13. AURKA is one of three related genes (AURKA, AURKB, and AURKC) encoding AURORA kinases/ serine-threonine kinases that play important roles in mitotic spindle formation and centrosome maturation and are physiologically essential for proper segregation of chromosomes into daughter cells.

Methods: To address its possibility as a therapeutic target for pancreatic cancer, we employed the RNA interference technique to knockdown AURKA expression and analyzed its phenotypes.

Results: We found that the specific knockdown of AURKA in cultured pancreatic cancer cells strongly suppressed in vitro cell growth and in vivo tumorigenicity. The knockdown induced the accumulation of cells in the G2/M phase and eventual apoptosis. Furthermore, we observed a synergistic enhancement of the cytotoxicity of taxanes, a group of chemotherapeutic agents impairing G2/M transition, by the RNA interference-mediated knockdown of AURKA.

Conclusions: These results indicate that inhibition of AURKA expression can result in potent antitumor activity and chemosensitizing activity to taxanes in human pancreatic cancer. In order to clarify the clinical implication of AURKA expression in pancreatic cancer tissues, we are now investigating the relationship between clinical data and the AURORA expression using immuno-staining study.

Clinical Acute Pancreatitis

80

Early Persistent Systemic Inflammatory Response Syndrome (SIRS) is Associated with the Severity of Multi-Organ Dysfunction (MOD) and Death from Acute Pancreatitis

R. Mofidi, M.D. Duff, S.J. Wigmore, K.K. Madhavan, O.J. Garden, R.W. Parks

Department of Clinical and Surgical Sciences, University of Edinburgh, UK

Aims: Mortality in patients with acute pancreatitis is associated with the number of failing organs and the severity and reversibility of organ dysfunction. The aim of this study was to assess the significance of early SIRS in the development of MOD and death from acute pancreatitis.

Methods: All patients with acute pancreatitis from January 2000 to December 2004 were reviewed. Serum C-reactive protein (CRP), APACHE II scores and presence of SIRS were recorded on admission and at 48-hours. Organ dysfunction scores were calculated during the first week of presentation. Presence of SIRS and elevated CRP levels on admission and 48-hours were correlated with the cumulative organ dysfunction scores in the first week. The association between persistent SIRS and death from acute pancreatitis was assessed.

Results: 759 patients with acute pancreatitis were identified of whom 45 (5.9%) died during the index admission. SIRS was identified in 162 patients on admission and 138 patients at 48 hours. The median cumulative MOD score in patients with persistent SIRS was significantly higher than in patients in whom SIRS resolved and patients with no SIRS [Median (range): 5 (0–12), 3 (0–7) and 0 (0–9) respectively, ($p < 0.001$)]. Thirty five patients (25.4%) with persistent SIRS died from acute pancreatitis compared with 5 patients (6.8%) with transient SIRS and 4 patients (0.7%) with no clinical evidence of SIRS in the first 48 hours of admission ($p < 0.001$). No correlation was observed between CRP levels on admission and MOD scores (p = ns), however there was a close correlation between CRP levels at 48 hours and MOD scores ($p < 0.001$).

Conclusions: Early SIRS is associated with MOD and death from acute pancreatitis. SIRS is a valuable bedside indicator of severity of acute pancreatitis during the first 48 hours of presentation.

81

Determinants of Survival following Surgery for Pancreatic Necrosis

R. Mofidi, S. Connor, S.J. Wigmore, K.K. Madhavan, O.J. Garden, R.W. Parks

Department of Clinical and Surgical Sciences, University of Edinburgh, UK

Aims: Infected pancreatic necrosis remains the major cause of delayed mortality from acute pancreatitis. This is treated by pancreatic necrosectomy which carries significant mortality. The aim of this study was to identify factors associated with mortality after pancreatic necrosectomy.

Methods: Patients who underwent pancreatic necrosectomy from January 1994 to December 2004 were reviewed. APACHE II scores, CRP levels, presence of systemic inflammatory response syndrome (SIRS) in the first 48 hrs were collected and multi-organ dysfunction (MOD) scores calculated. The association between these variables and mortality was assessed.

Results: 1,248 patients presented with acute pancreatitis of whom 94 (7.5%) underwent pancreatic necrosectomy (male: 51, female: 43). Median (range) age of the patients was 54 (21–80) years. Median APACHE II score on admission was 13 (5–22). Persistent SIRS was identified in 49 patients at 48 hours. The median cumulative MOD score was 2 (0–9) preoperatively and 4 (1–11) postoperatively. Twenty-three patients (24.5%) died. Those who died [Median age: 69 (40–80)] were older than survivors [Median age: 52 (19–79)], ($p < 0.05$) and had higher admission APACHE II scores [14 (12–19) vs. 9 (2–22)], ($p < 0.001$). There were significant associations between pre ($r^2 = 0.27$, $p < 0.01$) and postoperative ($r^2 = 0.3$, $p < 0.01$) MOD scores and mortality following pancreatic necrosectomy. Early SIRS ($p < 0.01$) and time between presentation and necrosectomy ($p < 0.01$) were independent predictors of survival. Pancreatic necrosectomy within 2 weeks of presentation was associated with significantly higher mortality [14/29 (48.2%)] than surgery after 2 weeks [9/65 (13.9%)], ($p < 0.01$).

Conclusions: Pancreatic necrosectomy carries higher mortality in patients with higher APACHE II scores, early SIRS and those with unresolved multi-organ dysfunction. Necrosectomy is associated with poorer outcome when performed within two weeks of presentation.

82

Removing of Pancreatic Ascites Ameliorates the Clinical Course of Necrotizing Pancreatitis

A. Perejaslov, S. Chooklin, R. Chukla

Medical University, Lviv, Ukraine

Introduction: Pancreatic ascites and fluid collections often accompanied the clinical course of severe acute pancreatitis. These fluid collections have no communications with the pancreatic ductal system and represent a serous or exudative reaction to the pancreatic inflammation and contain proteases, leukotrienes, cytokines, and others.

Methods: Levels of interleukins (IL) 6, 8, 17, and 18 in blood and fluid collections were measured, using the ELISA technique, in 31 patients with necrotizing pancreatitis. The percutaneous ultrasonic guided aspiration was applied in 20 patients with the limited fluid collections. The laparoscopic drainage was applied in 11 patients with the widespread pancreatic ascites. The control group compiled 12 patients without removing of fluid collections or pancreatic ascites.

Results: At the time of admission Ranson, APACHE II and Balthazar score, plasma levels of interleukins had no significant differences in both groups of patients. Besides that, the highest levels of interleukins were in exudate compared with plasma samples (IL-6 – 654.3 ± 29.2 vs. 603.5 ± 34.6 pg/ml; IL-8 – 327.3 ± 21.5 vs. 180.3 ± 22.3 pg/ml; IL-17 – 553.3 ± 79.8 vs. 372.1 ± 30.4 pg/ml; IL-18 – 696.0 ± 22.7 vs. 632.8 ± 25.2 pg/ml). Elimination of pancreatic ascites/fluid collections caused the decrease of interleukins concentration in plasma within first two days. The gradual increase of all interleukin levels up to the seventh day was noted in patients of the control group that accompanied with the progression of respiratory, cardiovascular insufficiency in 5 (41.7%) patients and necrotic changes in 7 (58.3%) patients. At the same time increase of Balthazar score was noted in 9 (29%) patients of the main group and progression of MODS in 4 (12.9%) patients ($p < 0.05$).

Conclusion: Thus, the removing of pancreatic ascites ameliorates the clinical course of necrotizing pancreatitis.

83

Hematologic Effects of Interleukin-17 in Acute Pancreatitis

S. Chooklin, A. Perejaslov

Medical University, Lviv, Ukraine

Introduction: Enhanced expression of cytokines often determined the severe course of acute pancreatitis, which characterized by the development of multiple organ dysfunction syndrome. IL-17 is a relatively recently described T-cell derived cytokine. Many of its effects are similar to, although in isolation less potent than, those of IL-1β and TNF-α. Thus, IL-17 may play an important role in acute pancreatitis.

Methods: Plasma levels of IL-17, using ELISA technique, were studied in 87 patients with acute pancreatitis who admitted in clinic within 48 hours after disease onset. According the Atlanta criterion the mild pancreatitis was established in 56 (64.4%) patients and 31 (35.6%) had necrotizing pancreatitis. The control group compiled 10 healthy volunteers.

Results: The IL-17 plasma level was detected only in one volunteer. The elevated IL-17 plasma levels were noted in all patients with acute pancreatitis, besides that, the highest levels were in patients with established severe pancreatitis (372.1 ± 83.3 vs. 162.8 ± 63.9 pg/ml, $p < 0.05$). The initial levels of IL-17 were higher in patients who subsequently developed purulent complications of severe pancreatitis but exceeding was insignificant. The gradual decrease of IL-17 levels were noted in all patients. The IL-17 levels clearly correlated with the quantity of total leukocyte, polymorphonuclear leukocytes and hemoglobin level at the time of admission. IL-17 has prominent proinflammatory properties due to the induction of numerous genes that are associated with inflammation, such as IL-1β, IL-6, TNF-α, and GM-CSF. Hematologic effects of IL-17 may be connected with its ability to induce the GM-CSF expression which is also enhanced in severe pancreatitis.

Conclusion: Thus, acute pancreatitis is accompanied by the rise in IL-17 plasma levels that correlated with the hematologic changes.

84

Use of Lanreotide in the Prevention of Pain Relapse following Reintroduction of Oral Diet in Patients following an Acute Episode of Acute Necrotizing Pancreatitis (ANP): Multicentre Prospective Randomized Placebo-Controlled Double-Blind Study

P. Lévy[1], T. Ponchon[2], P. Hastier[3], J. Sahel[4], A. Pariente[5], J.P. Arpurt[6], J. Escourrou[7], J. Boyer[8], A. Koch[9], G. Bommelaer[10], F. Paye[11], J.L. Porcheron[9], M. Bougeard-Julien[11], J. Blumberg[11], P. Ruszniewski[1]

Hospitals of [1]Clichy, [2]Lyon, [3]Nice, [4]Marseille, [5]Pau, [6]Avignon, [7]Toulouse, [8]Angers, [9]Paris, [10]Clermont-Ferrand, [11]Ipsen, Paris, France

Introduction: Rate of pain relapse at reintroduction of cyclic oral diet following an episode of ANP approaches 30% (Lévy et al. Gut 1997:262). Following lanreotide (open-labelled study, n = 23) in patients with ANP, pain relapse was only 4% (Lévy et al. Pancreatology 2004:229).

Aim: Evaluate lanreotide (30 mg i.m.) in prevention of pain-relapse at reintroduction of oral diet following ANP (double-blind randomised fashion).

Methods: Inclusion criteria: ANP defined as a Balthazar score ≥ D or 4 points, and pain-free without analgesics for at least 48 hrs. Clinical onset of non-complicated ANP < 30 days of enrollment. Lanreotide or placebo was injected 24 hrs before re-feeding (standardized). Randomization was stratified to the lipase level in the 24 hrs prior to re-feeding (±3 times normal [N]) (1). Judgement criterion was rate of pain relapse requiring interruption of oral feeding at 1 and 4 weeks.

Results: 77 patients were randomized (placebo, n = 39; lanreotide, n = 38). Both groups were comparable for age (median, 53 years), sex (M = 68%), chronic alcohol consumption (40%), chronic pancreatitis (5%), Ranson score ≥ 3 (16%), median CRP (225 mg/L), lipase ≤ 3N (74%), duration of pain (8-days) or fasting (10-days), enteral (8%) or parenteral nutrition (58%). More patients with Balthazar E scores were included in the placebo group (54 vs. 29%; $p < 0.03$). Medications were well-tolerated with no side effects. Only one patient (group lanreotide) experienced pain relapse at 7 days. One patient treated with lanreotide (3%) and 6 in the placebo group (15%) had pain relapse within 28 days ($p < 0.05$). Median hospitalization was 17 and 19 days in lanreotide and placebo groups, respectively (NS).

Conclusion: In the month following cyclic oral re-feeding in ANP, lanreotide significantly reduced pain relapse. Although this effect was not seen in the 1st week, lanreotide could prove efficacious in the prevention of pain relapse in such patients.

85

When and How to Refeed Acute Pancreatitis (AP) Patients? A Prospective, Randomized, Four-Way Study

J. Lariño-Noia, J. Iglesias-García, A. Villanueva-Rodríguez, J. Iglesias-Canle, M. Vilariño-Insua, M. Iglesias-Rey, J.E. Domínguez-Muñoz

Gastroenterology Department, University Hospital of Santiago de Compostela, Spain

Introduction: Oral feeding in AP is usually restarted by stepwise increase of caloric and fat intake once pain, fever, leucocytosis, ileus or a significant elevation of serum pancreatic enzymes are absent. The scientific evidence supporting this approach is however lacking. In the present study we tested the hypothesis that oral feeding in AP can be restarted as soon as ileus is absent and that a stepwise increase of the caloric intake is not required.

Patients and Methods: 39 consecutive patients (mean age 56 years, range 26–85 years, 18 male) diagnosed of AP were included in a prospective, open, randomized, four-way, comparative study. Two refeeding schedules (schedule A, stepwise caloric increase from 1207 kcal to 1767 kcal over 3 days; schedule B, initial diet containing 1767 kcal) and two oral refeeding times (early refeeding, as soon as ileus is absent; standard refeeding time, once pain, fever, leucocytosis, ileus and a significant hyperlipasemia are absent) were evaluated. Patients were randomly allocated to one of the following four groups: Group I (n = 12), schedule A at a standard refeeding time; group II (= 10), schedule A at an early refeeding time; group III (n = 9), schedule B at a standard refeeding time; and group IV (n = 8), schedule B at an early refeeding time. Tolerance to oral refeeding (main outcome) and the development of dyspeptic symptoms were evaluated. Intolerance was defined as AP relapse or severe pain, nausea or vomiting requiring interruption of oral feeding.

Results: All patients except two from group I tolerated oral refeeding. 14 patients (36%) developed dyspeptic symptoms (5 from group I, 2 from group II, 2 from group III and 5 from group IV), mainly postprandial fullness, which did not require the interruption of oral feeding.

Conclusion: Oral feeding in AP can be restarted with a 1,800 kcal, low fat diet. A careful stepwise increase of caloric intake is not needed. Absence of ileus but not of pain, leucocytosis, fever or elevation of serum pancreatic enzymes is required for oral feeding to be restarted.

86

Pancreatic Gene Expression for Markers in Human Pancreatitis

J. Bonior[1], J. Jaworek[1], D. Karcz[3], J. Panek[3], M. Tusiński[3], J. Zasada[3], S.J. Konturek[2], W.W. Pawlik[2]

[1]Department of Medical Physiology, Health Care Faculty, [2]Chair of Physiology, and [3]General Surgery II, Medical Faculty, Jagiellonian University School of Medicine, Cracow, Poland

Introduction: The severity of acute pancreatitis (AP) and multiorgan failure is correlated to the changes of the cytokine production and release. Melatonin and nitric oxide (NO) protects the pancreas against the damage in experimental models of AP. However the gene expression for cytokines nitric oxide synthase (NOS) or for L-tryptophan hydroxylase (HIOMT), an enzyme converting L-tryptophan into melatonin in human pancreas has not been presented yet. This study was undertaken to investigate the genes expression for inducible (iNOS) and constitutive (cNOS) forms of NO synthase and for pro-inflammatory interleukin 1β (IL-1β) and anti-inflammatory interleukin-10 (IL-10) in the human pancreatic tissue.

Methods: Pancreatic tissue samples were taken from 12 patients with necrotizing AP during surgery. Control samples were obtained from histologically unchanged pancreatic tissue obtained from 5 patients with pancreatic cancer. Gene expression for interleukins, cNOS, iNOS, and HIOMT was detected by RT-PCR. β-actin was determined in all samples as a housekeeping gene.

Results: HIOMT mRNA signal has been detected in the intact pancreas but was much stronger in all samples which were obtained from patients with necrotizing form of AP. Gene expression for cytokines (IL-1β, IL-10) and for iNOS , have been present in necrotizing pancreatitis, but not in the control pancreas, whereas mRNA signal for cNOS has been found in the control samples.

Conclusion: In humans, acute necrotizing pancreatitis resulted in the increase of pancreatic mRNA signals for iNOS, IL-1β, IL-10 and HIOMT.

87

The Imbalance between Matrix Metalloproteinase-9 and Tissue Inhibitor of Metalloproteinase-1 Concentrations in Patients with Acute Pancreatitis

U. Wereszczynska-Siemiatkowska[1], A. Dabrowski[1], A. Siemiatkowski[2], B. Mroczko[3], G. Sek[1]

[1]Department of Gastroenterology and Internal Medicine, [2]Anaesthesiology and Intensive Therapy, [3]Biochemical Diagnostics, Medical University of Bialystok, Poland

Introduction: In acute pancreatitis (AP) the balance between matrix metalloproteinases activity and their tissue inhibitors is an important factor providing extracellular matrix homeostasis. The aim of the study was to assess the metaloproteinase-9 (MMP-9) and its tissue inhibitor (TIMP-1) concentration profiles in serum of patients with AP depending on disease severity.

Methods: Prospective studies were performed in patients with mild (MAP, n = 18) and severe (SAP, n = 19) form of AP. Control comprised of 15 healthy volunteers.

Results: The serum MMP-9 concentration for the patients with MAP did not differ significantly from the values found in the healthy control. In the course of SAP, the serum MMP-9 concentration reached the highest values during the first three days of observation. At the day 1st, 2nd and 3rd it exceeded corresponding values for MAP, respectively by 283% ($p < 0.0001$), 194% ($p < 0.0001$) and 178% ($p < 0.0001$). Since the day 5th of SAP the decrease in MMP-9 concentration was observed. However, it still significantly exceeded the corresponding values found in MAP. The serum TIMP-1 concentration for both, patients with MAP and SAP was significantly higher than the values of the control group. In the course of the disease, TIMP-1 concentration in SAP was higher than in MAP and progressively increased until the day 5th. The significant correlation between MMP-9 and plasma concentration of polymorphonuclear leukocyte elastase (PMN-E) (Rs = 0.605, $p < 0.0001$) as well as serum concentration of C-reactive protein (Rs = 0.545, $p < 0.001$) was found. The significant correlation was also found between TIMP-1 and PMN-E (Rs = 0.415, $p < 0.01$) as well as between MMP-9 and TIMP-1 (Rs = 0.340, $p < 0.01$).

Conclusions: An early disturbance of the dynamic equilibrium between MMP-9 and TIMP-1 in severe AP may suggest that endogenous TIMP-1 is unable to balance the excessive activation and release of MMP-9. The MMP-9 may represent a new indicator of AP severity.

88

Prospective Randomized Double-Blind Placebo-Controlled Multicenter Trial of Glyceryl Nitrate Preventing Post-ERCP Pancreatitis

C. Nøjgaard[1], M. Hornum[2], S. Shulze[2], M. Elkjær[3], M. Kantowsky[3], P. Vilman[3], C. Jansen[4], A. Valkonen[5], L. Heyries[6], T. Hauge[7], K. Bakkevold[8], M.L. Skov[9], L.B. Svendsen[9], F. Møller Pedersen[10], O. Schaffalitzky de Muckadell[10], P. Matzen[1]

[1]Dept. of Gastroenterology, Hvidovre Hospital, Denmark, [2]Dept. of Internal Medicine and Surgery, KAS Glostrup, Denmark, [3]Dept. of Gastroenterology and Surgery D, KAS Gentofte, Denmark, [4]Dept. of Surgery, University Hospital Malmö, Sweden; [5]Tampere University Hospital, Finland; [6]Dept. of Gastroenterology, St Marguerite Hospital, Marseille, France; [7]Div. of Gastroenterology, Østfold County Hospital Fredrikstad, Norway; [8]Dept. of Surgery, Haugesund Hospital, Norway; [9]Dept. of Gastroenterological Surgery CTX, Rigshospitalet, Copenhagen, Denmark; [10]Dept. of Internal Medicine S, Odense University Hospital, Denmark

Introduction: Acute pancreatitis is the most common complication to an ERCP procedure. Although most episodes of post-ERCP pancreatitis (PEP) are mild, some patients develop severe necrotic pancreatitis resulting in prolonged hospitalization and significantly increased morbidity and mortality. Two studies have shown a significant effect of glyceryl nitrate (GN) preventing PEP. We wanted to evaluate this promising effect in a larger study with a more realistic precalculated incidence of PEP than the previous studies.

Methods: The trial is a randomized, double-blind placebo-controlled multicenter study including patients from six european countries. Other centers may be candidates for participation. The trial has started in October 2004. The number of patients necessary to decrease the frequency of PEP from 6% in the placebo-group to 3% in the GN-group is 1600 (α: 0.05, β: 0.20). The active drug is a patch containing 15 mg GN released over 24 hours and the placebo patch is a piece of Tegaderm. Primary endpoint is post procedure pancreatitis. Patients having this complication will be followed until recovery, death or steady state has been reached. Secondary endpoints are mild, moderate and severe pancreatitis, post procedure pancreatitis-related mortality, and adverse events.

Results: In February 2005, 77 patients have been included. F/m: 46/31, smokers/non-smokers: 34/42, median age: 69 (range 21–94), median alcohol intake: 2.5 g per week (range 0–650 g), median BMI: 24.9 (range 17.4–44.6). 6 patients have had PEP (7.8%), 1 mild, 4 moderate and 1 severe. One patient is dead after the procedure, as the result of liver metastasis. Three patients had headache and 2 hypotension.

Conclusion: The precalculated frequency (6.0%) of PEP is in accordance with the frequency (7.8%) in these preliminary data of the first 77 patients.

89

Prognostic Value of Sequential Organ Failure Assessment (SOFA) in Acute Pancreatitis

E. De Madaria[1], J. Martínez[1], Y. Calero[2], J. Sánchez-Payá[3], L. Sempere[1], M. Pérez-Mateo[2]

[1]Sección de Aparato Digestivo, [2]Servicio de Medicina Interna, [3]Servicio de Medicina Preventiva, Hospital General Universitario de Alicante, Spain

Introduction: Among the Atlanta criteria for definition of severe acute pancreatitis (SAP), the development of organ failure (OF) is thought to be the main factor related to mortality.

Aims: To evaluate the prognostic value of SOFA and the persistence of organic failure in patients with severe acute pancreatitis.

Methods: We include patients with AP. APACHE II and SOFA score were calculated daily during the first three days of admission. Severity of AP was assessed by Atlanta criteria. We used ROC curves to determine the cut off point of APACHE II with a NPV = 90%. According to this point, patients were divided into two groups: group A (APACHE II equal or above this cut off point) and group B (APACHE II below the cut off point). In each group, we evaluated the relationship between severity-mortality and persistence of OF (according to SOFA) during the three days.

Results: 137 patients were included (62 men; 21.2% SAP). The relationship between APACHE II and severity was significant in the three days evaluated. In the first day of admission (AUC: 0.734) the selected cut off point to achieve PNV of 90% was 4. In group A patients with persistent OF presented significantly SAP (51.9% vs. 22.2% in patients without or transient OF; p = 0.01) and mortality were also significantly higher (14.8% vs. 0%; p = 0.008). In group B only one patient developed complications and any died.

Conclusions: In our patients, APACHE II is a good prognostic factor but the cut off point with a high NPV seems too low. In the subgroup of patients with predicted SAP, monitoring SOFA allows to predict the development of complications and mortality, specially in patients with persistent OF.

90

Role of Endoscopic Ultrasound for the Diagnostis of Idiopathic Acute Pancreatitis: A Prospective Study Three Years after the French Consensus Conference

P. Andrau, B. Bournet, J. Moreau, J. Escourrou, L. Buscail

Department of Gastroenterology, CHU Rangueil, Toulouse, France

Introduction: The French consensus conference on acute pancreatitis (AP) in 2001 concluded that endoscopic ultrasound (EUS) was one of the best investigation to explore AP without evident cause after initial common investigations i.e. 'so called idiopathic AP' (IAP). According that, in our tertiary referral center, we prospectively evaluate over one year what was the real clinical impact of EUS performed at distance to an attack of IAP.

Patients and Methods: Between January and October 2004, 28 consecutive patients (M: 17, W: 11, mean age 48 years) with a recent IAP and referred in our center for bilio-pancreatic EUS were included. For each patient were recorded at time of EUS: time delay between AIP and EUS, investigation initially performed, daily alcohol consumption, serum phospho-calcium and glyco-lipidic parameters.

Results: Time delay between AIP and EUS was of 6.2 ± 2.2 weeks (4–12). All patients initially underwent CT scan, abdominal US. Balthazar score was: AB or C in 17 (61%), DE in 11 cases (39%). At time of EUS, new biological investigations were in the normal range and chronic alcohol consumption was definitively excluded. EUS was normal in 15 cases (true IAP) but revealed a cause in 13 patients (46.5%): gallbladder minilithiasis (n = 3) and sludge (n = 1) as well as early non calcified chronic pancreatitis (n = 9: idiopathic n = 7, autoimmune n = 2).

Conclusion: In all cases of IAP, EUS was performed according to the recommendations of French Consensus Conference 2001. In half of cases, EUS performed at distance, revealed a minilithiasis or an early chronic pancreatitis that had been not detected by initial standard investigations. The role of EUS in the diagnosis of IAP is strengthened by this prospective evaluation.

91

Continued Abuse Predicts Recurrent Acute Alcoholic Pancreatitis, but Metabolic Disorders May Be Involved

H. Pelli[1], R. Lappalainen-Lehto[1], A. Piironen[2], J. Sand[1], I. Nordback[1]

[1]Department of Gastroenterology and Alimentary Tract Surgery, [2]Department of Radiology, Tampere University Hospital, Finland

Introduction: Previously we showed in a retrospective study that 46% of the patients with acute alcoholic pancreatitis had a recurrent attack within 10–20 years. Young age and mild first pancreatitis predicted recurrences. The aim of this prospective study was to find risk factors for recurrences.

Patients and Methods: The patients surviving their first acute alcohol induced pancreatitis 1/2001 till 1/2003 were included. There were 57 patients (47 male and 10 female) with mean age of 45 (25–71) years. The diagnostic criteria for acute pancreatitis was epigastric pain, serum amylase $> 3 \times$ UNR, elevated serum CRP concentration consistent with signs of acute pancreatitis in abdominal imaging. Other aetiologies were excluded. Heavy alcohol consumption was detected by AUDIT. The endocrine and exocrine serum and faecal markers, alcohol consumption (grams) and secretin stimulated MRCP were performed to exclude morphological changes within four months after the hospitalization. The follow-up was mean 28 (12–48) months.

Results: 14 (24%) patients had a recurrent attack of acute alcoholic pancreatitis. In the univariate analysis higher body mass index (BMI) (28.0 vs. 25.5; $p = 0.01$), lesser amount of alcohol consumed before (AUDIT 20 vs. 25; $p = 0.03$) and after (512 g vs. 1260 g; $p = 0.004$) the first attack, and higher serum vitamin A concentration (3.3 μmol/l vs. 1.2 μmol/l; $p = 0.04$) were associated with lower risk of recurrence. Changes in secretin stimulated MRCP didn't correlate with recurrence. Age or severity of the first attack didn't predict recurrence. In the multivariate analysis the BMI was the only independent risk factor (OR = 0.82, 95% CI 0.69–0.99) indicating lower recurrence risk in more obese patients.

Conclusion: Heavy alcohol consumption before and continued abuse after the first acute pancreatitis is associated with recurrences, whereas morphological changes in pancreas seem to be less important. The possible association with metabolic disorders in recurrence warrants further investigation.

92

Is Acute Alcoholic Pancreatitis Part of Withdrawal Symptoms?

I. Nordback, H. Pelli, R. Lappalainen Lehto, J. Sand

Department of Gastroenterology and Alimentary Tract Surgery, Tampere University Hospital, Tampere, Finland

Background: Previously we have found that alcoholics develop pancreatic enzyme increases in serum during the withdrawal period even without clinical pancreatitis. Also in healthy young volunteers pancreatitis associated protein increases after, not during, the heavy alcohol consumption. In this study we investigated the time course of the development of the first symptoms of the first acute alcoholic pancreatitis in respect to stopping of alcohol consumption.

Methods: Early during the hospitalization, the first acute alcoholic pancreatitis patients (85 men, 15 women, 46 [18–73] years) were asked: Had you stopped continuous drinking already before the start of the acute abdominal pain later leading you to hospital? Had you stopped continuous drinking already before you started to feel nauseous or vomited? How many hours after the last drop of alcohol you started to feel pain (0 h, 1–6 h, 7–12 h, 13–24 h, 25–48 h, >48 h)? We assessed the amount of alcohol consumed in grams and the severity of the pancreatitis with serum C-reactive protein, pancreatic necrosis, pancreatic complications and the length of hospital and intensive care unit (ICU) stay.

Results: 85 patients responded. 91% developed nausea/vomiting and 69% pain not before they already had stopped drinking. Majority of the patients developed the symptoms during the first day of withdrawal (43%) or later (28%), mainly then during the second day. The timing of the symptoms was dependent both in the univariate analysis and in the multivariate analysis on the amount of alcohol consumed both during the past two months and the past week, but not on the severity of pancreatitis or the length of stay in hospital or in ICU.

Conclusions: In the majority of the patients with the first acute alcoholic pancreatitis the symptoms begin during the early withdrawal period. The withdrawal period might be more important than previously emphasized in the development of acute alcoholic pancreatitis.

93

Are beta-Lactams Better than Quinolones at Preventing Infection of Pancreatic Necrosis?

E.A. Villatoro[1], R.I. Hall[2], M. Larvin[1]

[1]Division of GI Surgery, University of Nottingham Medical School, Derby, UK, [2]Derby City General Hospital, Derby Hospitals NHS Trust, Derby, UK

Introduction: Controversy continues over efficacy of antibacterial therapy for preventing infection in pancreatic necrosis. Individual trials have been underpowered, and conflicting results leave clinicians confused. Meta-analysis suggested benefit, but interpretation was hindered by the variety of agents used.

Methods: The aim of the study was to determine whether the antibacterial agent used influences outcome. We sought randomised controlled trials (RCTs) comparing antibacterial therapy with placebo in patients with significant necrosis at CT. Five relevant RCTs were identified with regimens falling into two groups: three evaluated beta-lactams (n = 192), and two quinolone/imidazole (n = 102). None was adequately powered, and only one was double-blinded. Meta-analysis was performed using 'RevMan' software (Update, Oxon UK).

Results: Overall analysis (n = 294) suggested significantly less mortality with therapy (6%) versus controls (15.3%), odds ratio 0.37 (95% CI 0.17–0.83), however rates for infected necrosis were not significantly different. Prophylaxis with beta-lactams was associated with significantly less mortality (6.3%) than controls (16.6%), odds ratio 0.34 (95% CI 0.13–0.91), whereas there was no significant difference between quinolone/imidazole and controls. Beta-lactam treatment was associated with a significantly lower incidence of infected necrosis (15.6%) versus controls (29.2%), odds ratio 0.41 (95% CI 0.20–0.85), whilst there was no significant difference between quinolone/imidazole and controls. Similar results were observed for other end-points.

Conclusions: The results suggest that beta-lactams are efficacious whereas quinolone/imidazole regimens are not. This conflicts with tissue penetration studies, and suggests that antibacterial spectrum is more important than pharmacokinetics. Nevertheless, concerns persist about poor quality of studies, and a lack of data on adverse effects. Further, adequately powered, double-blinded studies of beta-lactam agents are urgently required to confirm efficacy and safety.

94

Role of Systemic Inflammatory Response Syndrome in the Relationship between Obesity and Severity of Acute Pancreatitis

L. Sempere[1], B. Lozano[1], J.M. Martínez[1], E. De Madaria[1], J. Sánchez-Payá[2], M.J. Poveda[1], M. Pérez-Mateo[1]

[1]Department of Gastroenterology and [2]Service of Preventive Medicine, Hospital General Universitario de Alicante, Alicante, Spain

Background: The inflammatory response plays a fundamental role in the clinical course of acute pancreatitis (AP). The obesity favours the development of local and systemic complications in AP, but the pathogenesis of this relationship remains unknown. Obese population may has a proinflammatory status which develops uncontrolled inflammatory cascade in patients with AP and obesity.

Aim: To assess the role of systemic inflammatory response in the relationship between obesity and severity of AP.

Patients and Methods: We collected prospectively patients admitted for AP in our hospital between February 2003 and May 2004. Anthropometric parameters and serum levels of IL-6 and IL-8 were determined within 48 hours of the AP beginning. Sex, age and BMI matched healthy controls were also considered. Obesity was defined as BMI $\geq$ 30 kg/m^2.

Results: A total of 85 patients with acute AP and 40 healthy controls were collected. The AP causes were biliary 67%, alcoholic 5.8%, idiopathic 17.6% and others 9.4%. Clinical course was severe in 22 (25.9%) patients. Serum levels of IL-6 and IL-8 in the total of persons studied were higher in obese persons than non-obese persons ($p = 0.09$; $p = 0.009$). In the AP group the obesity correlated with the severity of AP ($p = 0.047$) and serum level of IL-6 and IL-8 ($p = 0.027$; $p = 0.026$). We did not find differences in IL-6 and IL-8 between obese and non-obese healthy controls.

Conclusions: In obese patients, the increased incidence of severe AP is related to systemic inflammatory response.

95

Importance of Computed Tomography and Magnetic Resonance Imaging in the Assessment of Acute Pancreatitis

M. Radic[1], D. Miletic[2], D. Štimac[1], K. Baraba[1], D. Perkovic[1], S. Milic[1]

[1]Department of Gastroenterology, [2]Department of Radiology, Clinical Hospital Centre Rijeka, Rijeka, Croatia

Background and aims: Computed tomography (CT), especially a contrast-enhanced provides important information on the severity and prognosis of acute pancreatitis. Magnetic resonance imaging (MRI) has become a useful tool as an alternative to CT in assessment of acute pancreatitis. The aim of our study was to compare the diagnostic performance of MRI with CT in assessment of acute pancreatitis from third to fifth day after admission.

Patients and Methods: The study included 48 patients (23 males, 25 females, median age, 59 years; range 20–82) with diagnosis of acute pancreatitis admitted to our hospital during the period between January and September 2004. The inclusion criteria consisted of combination of clinical features, a typical case history, elevation of serum pancreatic enzymes and diagnosis confirmed by imaging studies. Contrast-enhanced spiral CT (Shimatzu, Japan) and MRI 0,5T (Shimatzu, Japan) exams were performed in all patients from third to fifth day after admission and Balthazar grade, extent of peripancreatic necrosis, CTSI (CT Severity index) and MRSI (MR Severity index) were calculated. In correlation assessment we used Spearman rank test.

Results: There is a correlation between spiral CT and MRI in evaluation of the inflammation extent, according to Balthazar ($r = 0.848$) and of severity according to Severity Index – SI ($r = 0.617$). In seven patients MRI showed hemorrhage that CT didn't reveal.

Conclusion: Diagnostic performance of CT and MRI in patients with acute pancreatitis doesn't differ significantly using Balthazar's grade, CTSI and MRSI. MRI is sensitive in diagnosing patients with hemorrhagic necrosis and can give additional information in that group of patients.

96

Serum Profile of IL-10 in Patients with Different Degrees of Acute Pancreatitis

J. Panek, J. Zasada, M. Dolecki, M. Tusiński, D. Karcz

2nd Surgical Department, College of Medicine, Jagiellonian University, Cracow, Poland

Background and aim: IL-10 is the most potent antiinflammatory cytokine. The aim of this study was to determinate the profile of IL-10 in serum of patients with different forms of acute pancreatitis (AP) during the first seven days of the treatment.

Methods: The study included 73 patients with mild AP and 28 patients with severe AP. Gallstones and alcohol were the two common causes of the disease (respectively: 56 and 45 patients) . Blood samples were taken on 1, 3, 5 and 7 days after admission to the hospital. Serum IL-10 was measured by using an ELISA kit (Biosource S.A.).

Results: At the admission the highest mean value for IL-10 was received from patients with severe biliary AP (28.6 pg/ml). On the following days the mean values of IL-10 systematically increased and on the 7th day reached 95.5 pg/ml. The mean values of IL-10 in patients with mild biliary form of the disease were: 10.5 pg/ml at the day of admission, and 5.3 pg/ml on the 7th day . The mean value of IL-10 in patients with alcoholic severe AP was slightly higher as compare to mild form (respectively: 21.2 and 19.2 pg/ml). In severe form of alcoholic AP on the last two days of analysis the mean values decreased (respectively: 18.3 and 15.6 pg/ml). The mean values in mild alcoholic form of AP during the next days rapidly decreased to 0.98 pg/ml (3rd day)and 0.5 pg/ml (5th day).

Conclusions: The serum levels of IL-10 were markedly elevated in severe AP at the day of admission. This level on the following days increased in severe biliary AP. In contrast, in severe alcoholic AP the mean level of IL-10 decreased and this phenomenon can indicate the disturbance of immune system in patients with alcoholic AP.

97

Systemic Endothelin-1 Concentrations Correlate with Severe Organ Failure and Multi Organ Dysfunction in Patients with Acute Pancreatitis

B.M. Rau[1], B. König[1], C.M. Krüger[1], M.K. Schilling[1], M. Bauer[2]

[1]Dept. of General- Visceral-, and Vascular Surgery, University of the Saarland, Homburg/Saar, Germany and [2]Dept. of Anesthesiology and Intensive Care Medicine, University of Jena, Germany

Introduction: Endothelin-1 (ET-1), a potent vasoconstrictor is thought to play a major role in mediating local and systemic severity in experimental acute pancreatitis (AP) by impairing microcirculation. However, clinical data on the course of Endothelin-1 in patients with AP are scarce.

Patients and Methods: We included 49 patients with AP in the present study. Necrotizing pancreatitis (NP) was present in 29 (59%) patients of whom 16 (55%) developed pancreatic infections. Systemic complications in terms of pulmonary failure, renal failure, and shock were observed in 67%, 35%, and 39% of all patients, respectively. Multi organ dysfunction syndrome (MODS) involving all three organ systems was found in 52% of patients with NP. The 38 amino acid ET-1 precursor big ET-1 was measured daily over two weeks after admission by a commercially available ELISA in EDTA plasma previously sampled and stored at –70°C.

Results: Big ET-1 concentrations were significantly increased in patients who developed pancreatic infections compared to patients with sterile necrosis or edematous pancreatitis. In contrast, the presence or absence of pancreatic necrosis had only little influence on big ET-1 levels. As far as systemic complications are concerned, systemic big ET-1 release was most expressed in patients with severe organ failure requiring ICU support such as mechanical ventilation, dialysis/hemofiltration, or pressure support, and in patients who developed MODS. By receiver-operating characteristics (ROC) analysis the closest correlation was found between maximum big ET-1 concentrations and the development of severe pulmonary failure and shock.

Conclusions: Our clinical data support previous experimental observations that Endothelin-1 plays a detrimental role in the pathogenesis of severe organ failure and MODS in AP.

98

Assessment of Major Complications and Overall Prognosis by the SOFA, APACHE II and MOF Score in Severe Acute Pancreatitis: Results of an International Multicenter Study

B.M. Rau[1], E. Kemppainen[2], C. Bassi[3], W. Uhl[4], M.W. Büchler[4], P. Puolakkainen[2], H.G. Beger[5], M.K. Schilling[1]

[1]Dept. of General, Visceral, and Vascular Surgery, Univ. of the Saarland, Homburg/Saar, Germany; [2]Dept. of Surgery, Helsinki University Central Hospital, Helsinki, Finland; [3]Dept. of Surgery and Gastroenterology, Pancreatic Unit, Univ. of Verona, Italy; [4]Dept. of Visceral- and Transplantation Surgery, Univ. of Bern, Switzerland; [5]Dept. of General Surgery, Univ. of Ulm, Germany

Introduction: Dynamic multiple parameter scoring systems are an established means for a fast and easy severity assessment in acute pancreatitis (AP). However, their role in predicting major complications or overall prognosis in severe AP has not been sufficiently validated yet.

Patients and Methods: A total of 104 patients with severe AP were included in five European centers within 96 hours of disease onset. CT-proven pancreatic parenchymal necrosis was present in 72 (69%) patients, 17 (16%) patients developed infected necrosis (IN). Multiple organ dysfunction syndrome (MODS) was present in 28 (27%) patients, and 8 patients (8%) died. Sequential organ failure assessment (SOFA), APACHE II, and multiple organ failure (MOF/Goris) scores were determined daily over a maximum of 21 days.

Results: Receiver-operating characteristic (ROC) analysis was based on the two highest values of each scoring system within the total observation period as well as on the values at 48 hours after disease onset. The results are shown below:

		Cut-Off	Sensitivity	Specificity
Prediction of death	SOFA max	> 7	88%	87%
	SOFA 48 h	> 4	86%	79%
	APACHE II max	> 20	88%	98%
	APACHE II 48 h	> 15	67%	90%
	MOF max	> 3	94%	79%
	MOF 48 h	> 3	100%	85%

The assessment of MODS or severe infected necrosis was possible with similar sensitivity and specificity rates. No statistical difference was found between the three scoring systems.

Conclusion: Each of the three scoring-systems allows an early and reliable assessment of major complications as well as overall prognosis in severe AP. Comprising fewer variables SOFA and MOF scores are easier to calculate than the APACHE II system while reaching at least the same diagnostic accuracy.

Bacterial infection and extend of necrosis has a strong impact on the occurrence of organ failure in NP. Future therapeutic strategies should be reduction of systemic complications by decreasing the rate of infected pancreatic necrosis or by impact on pathophysiological pathways responsible for development of organ failure.

99

Combination of Early Nasojejunal Feeding with Modern Synbiotic Therapy in the Treatment of Severe Acute Pancreatitis (Prospective, Randomized, Double-Blinded Study)

A. Oláh, T. Belágyi, Á. Issekutz

Department of Surgery, Petz Aladár Teaching Hospital, Györ, Hungary

Background: We and others showed previously that probiotics containing lactobacilli significantly improve the outcome of acute pancreatitis. 'Synbiotic 2000', a new synbiotic composition with high colony forming unit (CFU) comprises four different types of pre- and probiotics. In this prospective, randomized, double-blinded study we evaluated the role of 'Synbiotic 2000' in the treatment of severe acute pancreatitis.

Methods: Patients with severe acute pancreatitis were randomized into two groups. Nasojejunal feeding was commenced within 24 hours after admission in both groups and continued for at least seven days. The first group of patients received four different lactobacilli preparations with 10^{10} CFU, respectively, and prebiotics containing four bioactive fibers (inulin, beta-glucan, resistant starch and pectin) in addition. Patients in the second (control) group received only prebiotics.

Results: 62 patients with severe acute pancreatitis completed the study. Altogether 8 patients died. We detected lower incidence of multiorgan failure (MOF), septic complications and mortality in the first group compared to the control, but the differences were not significant statistically. The total incidence of systemic inflammatory response syndrome (SIRS) and MOF were significantly different between the two groups (8 vs. 14; $p < 0.05$). Furthermore, the number of patients recovering with complications were significantly less in the first group receiving modern synbiotic therapy compared to the control ($p < 0.05$). Finally, we found a lower rate of late (over 48 hours) organ failure in the first versus the control group (3.0% vs. 17.2%).

Conclusion: Our results suggest that early nasojejunal feeding with synbiotics may prevent organ dysfunctions in the late phase of severe acute pancreatitis. In addition, our data also indicate that the infection of pancreatic necrosis may be associated with early phase organ failure.

100

Acute Pancreatitis during Dialysis Treatment: more Frequent and Severe in Peritoneal than in Haemodialysis Patients

P.G. Lankisch[1], B. Weber-Dany[1], P. Maisonneuve[2], A.B. Lowenfels[3]

[1]Municipal Clinic of Lueneburg, Germany; [2]European Institute of Oncology, Milan, Italy; [2]New York Medical College, Valhalla, NY, USA

Introduction: The suggestion that acute pancreatitis (AP) may occur during dialysis treatment and is more frequent after peritoneal dialysis (PD) than during hemodialysis (HD; Gut 2001;46:385–289) was questioned.

Patients and Methods: A questionnaire was sent out to 1150 dialysis centers in Germany, asking for the incidence and severity of a first attack of AP, in 2002. Parameters of severity were serum amylase/lipase levels <3 the upper limit of normal (N), severe abdominal pain, signs of peritonitis, abnormal ultrasound and/or contrast-enhanced computed tomography, presence of pancreatic necrosis and an indication for hospital admission.

Results: 832 centers (response rate 72%) reported 46 HD-AP patients out of a total of 68,716 HD-patients (incidence rate 0.07, 95% confidence interval 0.05–0.09%) and 10 PD-AP patients out of a total of 3,386 PD-AP (0.30%, 0.15–0.57%, $p < 0.001$). When patients with idiopathic AP only were considered and those with AP due to alcohol abuse, biliary disease and other etiologies were excluded, the incidence rates were 0.03%, 0.02–0.05% and 0.12, 0.04–0.33%, $p = 0.03$. The rate of AP per 100,000 inhabitants/year was 78 for all AP-patients and 67 and 295 for HD and PD-AP-patients, respectively. These results were distinctly higher than those reported for the population in Lueneburg County (20, Pancreatology 2002;2:469–477). Patients on PD were more likely to have used medication responsible for the induction of drug-induced AP. They were also more likely to experience the onset of symptoms during dialysis ($p = 0.028$), a serum lipase >3N ($p = 0.074$) and have necrotizing AP ($p = 0.16$). Finally, they required hospitalisation more frequently.

Conclusion: A first attack of AP in dialysis patients occurs more frequently than in the general population and is more frequent and tends to be more severe in PD than in HD patients. Gastroenterologists, who are asked to see dialysis patients with unexplained abdominal pain, should be aware of this.

101

Low Mortality with Early FNA and Aggressive Necrosectomy in Patients with Severe Necrotising Pancreatitis

T. Satyadas, Y. Habbab, T. Groot Wassink, E. McIntosh, D.M. Rae, M. Sinclair

Eastern Hepatobiliary Pancreatic Unit, Ipswich Hospital, Ipswich, UK

Aim: To assess whether early FNA for bacteriology followed by a policy of aggressive necrosectomy results in a low mortality in patients with necrotising pancreatitis.

Methods: Prospective data were collected on 76 consecutive patients with proven severe acute pancreatitis managed on our intensive care unit from February 1997 to March 2004. A policy of early CT scanning with FNA for bacteriology (FNAB) was adopted if pancreatic necrosis was evident. If FNAB was positive, pancreatic necrosectomy was carried out and retroperitoneal irrigation established. We collected data on severity scores, APACHE-II, CRP, morbidity and mortality. The main outcome measure was mortality.

Results: Of the 76 patients managed in ITU, 17 underwent necrosectomy. Only two deaths were recorded in the group undergoing surgery translating to a mortality rate of 11.8%.

Conclusions: Early FNAB combined with a policy of aggressive necrosectomy in FNAB positive cases results in low mortality in patients with necrotising pancreatitis.

Clinical Chronic Pancreatitis

102

Capabilities of Ultrosound Histography in Diagnostics of Different Clinicopathogenetic Variants of Chronic Alcoholic Pancreatitis

Y.A. Zagorenko, N.B. Gubergrits

Chair of the Internal Diseases, Donetsk State Medical University, Ukraine

Introduction: Chronic alcoholic pancreatitis (CAP) – most common ethiologic variant of chronic pancreatitis. But it may have different clinical manifestations in particular patients. Different clinicopathogenetic CAP variants require differential approaches to treatment. So we decided to work out differential diagnostic criterion for main variants of CAP on the basis of pancreas ultrasound histography.

Methods: 92 CAP patients were observed in our clinic. We used cluster method in assessment of clinical, laboratory, immunogenetic and sonographic data. This allowed to determine 2 variants of CAP: infiltrative-parenchymatous (152 patients) and indurative-fibrous (40 patients). Sonography and determination of ultrasound histogram in the region of pancreatic head was conducted with the help of apparatus ALOKA SSD 630. Using data of ultrasound histography we worked out an index (I), which numerator contains width of pancreas ultrasound histogram basis (B), denominator – the sum of initial interval (S – distance between levels of grey equal 1 and corresponding to first histogram elements) and histogram L index: $I = B/(S + L)$.

Results: Immunologic testing allowed to determine, that first variant of CAP is characterized by presence of HLA haplotype A10-Cw6 and antigens B18, DRB1*11; the second one – by presence of HLA antigens B13, B27, Bw40, DRB1*13. Patients with infiltrative-parenchymatous CAP had I index between 1.81–2.03 and in all cases it was higher than 1.80. In indurative-fibrous CAP – from 0.33 to 0.51 and I index was less than 0.52. Sensitivity of the ordinary pancreas sonography in diagnostics of infiltrative-parenchymatous CAP was 68.0%, indurative-fibrous CAP – 70.3%. The same in case of calculating I index – 97.5% and 100.0% correspondingly.

Conclusion: I index based on data of ultrasound histography of the pancreas let to increase the informative capacity of sonography in CAP diagnostics and to conduct differentiation between main clinicopathogenetic variants of the disease.

103

Comparison of Histology and Extracellular Matrix between Autoimmune and Alcoholic Chronic Pancreatitis

M.H. Kim[1], M.H. Song[1], S.J. Jang[2], S.K. Lee[1], S.S. Lee[1], D.W. Seo[1]

Departments of [1]Internal Medicine and [2]Pathology, University of Ulsan, College of Medicine, Asan Medical Center, Seoul, Korea

Introduction: In autoimmune chronic pancreatitis (AIP), the histology is known to be characteristic and histologic recovery including pancreatic fibrosis has been reported after steroid therapy. The aims of this study were to demonstrate whether these histologic findings were unique to AIP and evaluate any differences in the composition of extracellular matrix between AIP and ordinary chronic pancreatitis.

Methods: Histologic findings and extracellular matrix proteins (collagen types I, III, and IV and fibronectin) were evaluated in 15 patients with clinically proven AIP and compared with those of 8 patients with surgically treated alcoholic chronic pancreatitis (ACP).

Results: The pattern of fibrosis was mainly loose fibrosis with stromal edema in AIP, while it was dense fibrosis in ACP. Acinar atrophy was more diffuse and severe in AIP than ACP. While diffuse inflammation with same stage of inflammatory activity was observed in AIP, multifocal inflammation with different stage of inflammatory activity was seen in ACP. For extracellular matrix proteins, dense deposition (compared with normal controls) of collagen type III was observed more frequently in ACP than AIP ($p < 0.05$). ACP showed decreased deposition of collagen type IV more frequently than AIP ($p = 0.001$).

Conclusion: Fibrosis and inflammation are common to both AIP and ACP, but the pattern is very different between the 2 groups, and the deposition of collagen types III and IV is substantially different between AIP and ACP.

104

Transforming Growth Factor beta and Interleukin-8 in Patients with Chronic Pancreatitis

I. Bihalskyy, A. Perejaslov, S. Chooklin

Medical University, Lviv, Ukraine

Introduction: Transforming growth factor (TGF)-β_1 is a pluripotent growth factor and cytokine which is a major regulator of fibrogenesis and participates in the healing process, directing the migration of monocytes and fibroblasts. Interleukin (IL)-8 is a CXC-chemokine which is a potent neutrophils and macrophages attractant. Fecal elastase 1 and bicarbonate concentration are the markers of pancreatic exocrine insufficiency.

Methods: TGF-β_1, IL-8 plasma levels and faecal elastase 1 (E1) were studied, using the ELISA technique, in 42 patients with chronic relapsing pancreatitis. The bicarbonate concentration was also determined in these patients. The control group compiled 15 healthy volunteers.

Results: The elevated levels of TGF-β_1 were detected in 37 (88.1%) of patients with chronic pancreatitis while in the control group it was detected only in 13.3% of cases. The IL-8 levels were also significantly higher in patients with chronic pancreatitis than in the control group ($p < 0.05$). Impaired exocrine function (E1 $< 200\,\mu g/g$, bicarbonate concentration < 70 mEq/L) was found in 54.8% of patients and exocrine insufficiency (E1 $< 100\,\mu g/g$, bicarbonate concentration < 50 mEq/L) in 42.9% of patients. There was a clear correlation between the plasma levels of TGF-β_1, IL-8 and the degree of exocrine function disorders. Increased TGF-β_1 levels reflect the degree of the pancreatic tissue damage and IL-8 mediated the additional pancreatic injury due to the recruitment of neutrophils and macrophages.

Conclusion: Our results suggest that TGF-β_1 and IL-8 play an important role in the pathogenesis of exocrine insufficiency in patients with chronic relapsing pancreatitis.

105

Organ-Preserving Resection of the Pancreatic Head in Patients with Chronic Pancreatitis: a Five-Year Experience

G. Farkas, L. Leindler, G. Farkas Jr., M. Daróczi

Department of Surgery, University of Szeged, Faculty of Medicine, Szeged, Hungary

Introduction: In chronic pancreatitis (CP), enlargement of the pancreatic head develops in consequence of inflammatory alterations. This report is concerned with the organ-preserving pancreatic head resection (OPPHR), and results attained with this operation in a five years period.

Methods: In 110 patients (m: 82, f: 28; mean age: 47.5 yr.), OPPHR was performed. The preoperative morbidity comprised frequent abdominal pain, a weight loss in all patients, jaundice in 9 patients, and latent and insulin-dependent diabetes mellitus in 11 and 15 patients, respectively. The surgical procedure consists in a wide excision of the inflammatory tumour in the region of the pancreatic head, without division and cutting of the pancreas over the portal vein. Reconstruction, with drainage of the secretion from the remaining pancreas into the intestinal tract, takes place through a jejunal Roux-en-Y loop. In 9 icteric cases and in 14 patients with stenosis of the common bile duct, prepapillary bile duct anastomosis was also performed with the jejunal loop.

Results: Only one reoperation was performed in consequence of anastomosis bleeding, but no mortality was noted in the postoperative period. The duration of hospitalization ranged between 7 and 12 days. In the mean follow-up period of 2.5 years (range 0.5 to 5.0), 100 patients became complaint-free, 10 patients had moderate symptoms and the weight increased with a median of 10.4 kg (range 4–28). After one and two years of operation bilio-digestive anastomosis was performed in 4 patients in consequence of bile duct stenosis. No change was noted in the preoperative endocrine function of 104 patients but 6 patients with latent diabetes mellitus became IDDM.

Conclusions: The five-year experience reveals that this organ-preserving pancreatic head resection is an effective procedure for definitive control of the complications of CP.

106

Chronic Pancreatitis in Children – Single Center Experience

G. Oracz[1], B. Oralewska[1], M. Teisseyre[1], A. Sobczynska-Tomaszewska[2], J. Pertkiewicz[3], J. Ryzko[1], J. Bal[2], J. Socha[1]

[1]Department of Gastroenterology, Hepatology and Immunology, The Children's Memorial Health Institute, Warsaw, Poland, [2]Department of Medical Genetics, National Research Institute of Mother and Child, Warsaw, Poland, [3]Olympus Endotherapy, Warsaw, Poland

Introduction: Chronic pancreatitis is a rare disease in childhood. The etiology of chronic pancreatitis in children is varied and includes anatomic anomalies, gene mutations, metabolic disorders and others. The aim of this study was to evaluate etiological aspects of chronic pancreatitis in children.

Methods: Children with chronic pancreatitis hospitalized since 1995 to 2005 were enrolled into the study. Clinical and epidemiological data were recorded and analyzed. All children were screened for gene mutations by direct DNA sequencing. Imaging studies (ERCP, MRCP, CT) were performed in all children.

Results: 107 children with chronic pancreatitis were hospitalized. Mean age was 8.87 years (range : 2.0 to 19.4 years). Gene mutations were found in 34 children (32%) (PRSS1 mutation in 14 children, CFTR in 9 patients, SPINK1 in 16 children). In 6 cases two gene mutations were found. Hyperlipemia was found in 20 patients (18.7%). Sixteen patients (15%) had anatomic anomalies (13 pancreas divisum, 2 ansa pancreatica, 1 two main pancreatic ducts). chronic pancreatitis was associated with biliary disease in 10 patients (9.3%). History of trauma was present in 5 cases (4.7%). In 13 children we found autoantibody (12%). In two cases chronic pancreatitis was probably associated with neurological drugs, in 4 with lambliosis, in 1 with dermatomiositis, in 1 with colitis ulcerosa and in one with ascariasis. In 18 children we found more than one etiological factor (16.8%).

Conclusions: (1) The most common causes of chronic pancreatitis are gene mutations, metabolic disorders and anatomic anomalies. (2) Our data demonstrate the need for genetic testing in children with chronic pancreatitis. (3) We should be aware of coexisting etiologic factors causing chronic pancreatitis in children.

Support from research grant KBN 2P05E 10128.

107

What is the Natural History of Cystic Dystrophy of Aberrant Pancreas (CDAP)?

V. Rebours[1], P. Lévy[1], M.-P. Vullierme[2], A. Sauvanet[1], D. O'Toole[1], A. Aubert[1], L. Palazzo[1], F. Maire[1], P. Hammel[1], V. Vilgrain[2], J. Belghiti[1], P. Ruszniewski[1]

[1]Medical-Surgical Federation of Hepato-Gastroenterology, [2]Department of Radiology, Beaujon Hospital, AP-HP, University Paris VII, Clichy, France

Introduction: Natural history of CDAP and association with chronic calcified pancreatitis (CCP) is unknown. Imaging procedures (CT, EUS) allow preoperative diagnosis.

Aim: Describe clinical and morphological characteristics of CDAP in a large medicosurgical series.

Methods: All patients with CDAP diagnosed on CT and EUS (1995–2004) were consecutively included. Diagnosis: association of localised thickening of the GI wall (without destruction of wall layers) in the presence of $\geq$1 cyst within the submucosa or muscularis propria.

Results: 109 patients were studied (men: 90%; chronic alcoholism: 86%). Median age at 1st sign was 45 years. CCP was found in 69%. Main symptoms (% with/without CCP) were: pancreatic pain (92/79%; NS), weight loss (80/82%; NS; median loss, 16%), acute pancreatitis (49/35%; NS); vomiting (30/26%; NS); diabetes (45/15%; $p < 0.004$); steatorrhoea (28/9%, $p < 0.05$); jaundice (13/12%; NS); GI bleeding (1/12%; NS). Biological signs of inflammation and cholestasis occurred in 41% and 37%, respectively. CDAP involved the gastric antrum (9%), duodenum (96%; of which 91% involved the 2nd duodenum and duodeno-pancreatic side in 67%), and jejunum (1%). The majority of patients had $\geq$2 cysts (median diameter: 15 mm). Peri-duodenal inflammation and calcifications were observed in 47% and 11%, respectively. EGD (n 8 0) revealed: stenosis (52% (complete 6%), thickened folds (64%), normal (36%). No treatment was required in 20%. Specific treatment included: symptomatic (analgesics, gastric aspiration and artificial nutrition) in 80%; somatostatin analogues in 8%; endoscopic 15%; surgery (for GI stenoses or painful inflammatory mass) in 27% (Whipple's: 17, by-passes: 8).

Conclusion: CDAP occurs in men with chronic alcoholism and without CCP in 1/3 of cases. Apart from pancreatic exocrine insufficiency, symptoms (pain, acute pancreatitis, weight loss) are not different in patients with or without CCP. It most frequently involves the internal portion of the 2nd duodenum and cysts are usually small. Adapted surgery is required in only 1/3 of patients.

108

The Change of Resting Energy Expenditure in Patients with Decompensated Stage of Chronic Pancreatitis after Replacement Therapy by Pancreatic Enzyme and Insulin

M. Yanagimachi[1], Y. Tando[1], E. Shizuno[1], Y. Matsuhashi[1], A. Matsumoto[1], H. Tanaka[1], Y. Ogawa[1], T. Suda[1], T. Nakamura[2]

[1]Third Department of Internal Medicine, [2]Department of Health Science, Hirosaki University School of Medicine, Hirosaki, Japan

Introduction: Chronic pancreatitis is characterized by an evolution toward destruction of pancreas. As pancreatic insufficiency causes malnutrition, the assessment of resting energy expenditure (REE) is useful for nutritional support. The present study was undertaken to determine how changed the REE in patients with decompensated stage of chronic pancreatitis (DCP) after the replacement therapy by pancreatic enzyme and insulin.

Methods: The nutritional state and blood glucose profile were examined in 11 DCP patients, 10 diabetic patients with insulin defficiency and 10 healthy subjects. Eleven DCP patients consisted of 6 patients with normoalbuminemia (over 3.5 g/dl: group A), and 5 patients with hypoalbuminemia (under 3.5 g/dl: group B). REE was measured by indirect calorimetry (Metavine-N, Vine Bio-Dynamic Systems, Inc. Tokyo, Japan). Predicted energy expenditure (PEE) was calculated using the Harris-Benedict formula.

Results: The basal REE was higher in both DCP patients and diabetic patients than in healthy subjects. In DCP patients the basal REE was lower in group B (1148.1 $\pm$ 160.3 kcal) than in group A (1312.5 $\pm$ 252.3 kcal). After replacement therapy the REE was increased in 5 patients and decreased in 6 patients. On the other hand, the REE was decreased and equalled to PEE (REE/PEE: 1.0 $\pm$ 0.2) after insulin therapy for diabetic patients.

Conclusions: The REE was increased under the insulin deficiency. But when malnutrition has been continued long term in DCP patients, the REE was tended to decrease. The change of REE after replacement therapy for DCP patients will be affected by other factor except blood glucose profile and maldigestion.

109

Optimization of the Administration Schedule of Oral Pancreatic Enzyme Supplements in Patients with Exocrine Pancreatic Insufficiency: A Randomized, Three-Way, Crossover Study

J.E. Domínguez-Muñoz[1], J. Iglesias-García[1], M. Iglesias-Rey[1], A. Figueiras[2], M. Vilariño-Insua[1]

Departments of [1]Gastroenterology and [2]Clinical Epidemiology, University Hospital of Santiago de Compostela, Spain

Introduction: Oral pancreatic enzymes for the treatment of exocrine pancreatic insufficiency should be properly administered to optimize gastric mixture and emptying with the food. We aimed at assessing the efficacy of a portioned administration of oral pancreatic enzymes along meals in comparison to a single intake just before or just after meals in the treatment of exocrine pancreatic insufficiency.

Methods: A prospective, randomized, open, comparative, crossover study of three different administration schedules of oral pancreatic enzymes was carried out in 24 consecutive chronic pancreatitis patients with maldigestion secondary to exocrine pancreatic insufficiency. Four capsules containing 10,000 U lipase each in form of enteric-coated mini-microspheres (Kreon®, Solvay Pharma, Germany) were randomly given just before meals (schedule A), just after meals (schedule B) or distributed along meals (schedule C) during three consecutive one-week periods. Fat digestion before and on the last day of each one of the three treatment periods was evaluated by an optimized mixed ^{13}C-triglycerides breath test. The cumulative recovery rate of $^{13}CO_2$ was considered as the result of the test.

Results: Before therapy, the $^{13}CO_2$ recovery rate during the breath test was 23.8 ± 15.8% (normal >57.0%). The efficacy of oral pancreatic enzymes for improving fat digestion tended to be higher when capsules were taken along meals ($^{13}CO_2$ recovery 61.4 ± 21.4%) or just after meals ($^{13}CO_2$ recovery 60.6 ± 21.8%) than when taken just before meals ($^{13}CO_2$ recovery 53.9 ± 20.3%) ($p = 0.1$). The percentage of patients that normalized fat digestion under therapy was 50%, 54% and 63% with schedules A, B and C, respectively. Thus 13% and 9% more patients normalized fat digestion with schedule C than with schedules A and B, respectively.

Conclusion: The efficacy of pancreatic enzyme supplements for the treatment of exocrine pancreatic insufficiency may be optimized by a portioned administration of the capsules along meals.

110

Ultra Thin Needle Histology May Have a Role in Diagnosing Chronic Pancreatitis

J. Sand[1], A. Välikoski[1], T. Tani[2], J. Laukkarinen[1], J. Isola[2], I. Nordback[1]

[1]Department of Gastroenterology and Alimentary Tract Surgery, and [2]Department of Pathology, Tampere University Hospital, Tampere, Finland

Introduction: Diagnosis of chronic pancreatitis (CP) is based on symptoms, ductal or parenchymal changes in imaging studies, function tests and histology. Especially the diagnosis of mild CP is difficult. Pancreatic core biopsies might be associated with significant complication rate at least in normal pancreas, but fine needle aspiration techniques are widely used during endoscopic ultrasound. Our aim was to evaluate the accuracy of ultra thin needle histology, the needle size being the same as in aspiration biopsies, in the diagnosis of CP, having the histology of a large surgical biopsy as the 'golden standard' reference.

Methods: There were 50 patients; age 60 (28–82) yrs, who underwent pancreatic resection for any reason. Two needle biopsies (outer diameter of 0.8 mm, study biopsies) and a 5 × 5 mm piece of tissue (reference biopsies) were taken from the same site of the specimen avoiding suspected neoplastic areas in the specimen. The samples were analysed for inflammation and fibrosis, both graded 0–3, as well as for any neoplastic changes without knowing the medical history, operative findings or final histology.

Results: The reference biopsy showed normal tissue in 19 (38%), CP in 29 (58%) and only mild fibrosis (grade 1) in 2 (4%) patients. In one patient the needle biopsy was insufficient for analysis. There was an agreement between ultra thin needle histology and control specimen in 45/49 (92%) patients (correlation coefficient 0.9). Two CP and one mild inflammation were misclassified as normal tissue (these patients didn't have any clinical symptoms or signs of CP in imaging), while 1 CP was misclassified as adenocarcinoma. Sensitivity of needle biopsy for CP was 89% and specificity was 100%. The grade of inflammation and fibrosis were under estimated in needle histology in 16% and 18%, respectively, and they both were over estimated in 8% when compared to wedge biopsy.

Conclusions: Ultra thin needle histology correlates well with pancreatic wedge biopsy. Thus, its role in diagnosing various grades of chronic pancreatitis needs to be studied.

111

Unexpected Low Common Occurrence of Chronic Pancreatitis and Alcoholic Liver Disease

J. Spicak[1], P. Poulova[1], T. Hucl[1], P. Trunecka[1], J. Sperl[1], P. Taimr[1], P. Drastich[1], M. Ryska[2], M. Oliverius[2]

[1]Department of Hepatogastroenterology, [2]Department of Surgery, Institute for Clinical and Experimental Medicine, Prague, Czech Republic

Background and Aim: Alcohol is a frequent cause of liver cirrhosis and a dominant cause of chronic pancreatitis. The aim of this study was to assess the common occurrence of both these diseases.

Methods: Since the year 2000, we have evaluated I: 421 patients with liver cirrhosis who underwent comprehensive examination with the aim to assess their ability to have liver transplantation (group I), and II: 136 patients primarily managed for chronic pancreatitis (group II).

Results: Group I: Chronic pancreatitis was diagnosed in 12 (2.9%) patients with alcoholic liver cirrhosis. The mean age at the time of diagnosis of pancreatitis was 42.8 years. In one patient, a biliary stent was implanted while two required pancreatic surgery. Two patients with chronic pancreatitis underwent liver transplantation. Group II: Of the 136 patients with chronic pancreatitis, liver cirrhosis was diagnosed in 27 (19.9%), being due to cholestasis (bile duct stenosis) in 2 and to alcoholic liver damage in 25. Esophageal varices were found in 20 patients, out of which number in 7, the varices were due to prehepatic portal hypertension. Overall, common occurrence of liver cirrhosis and chronic pancreatitis was demonstrated in 39 (7%) of the 557 patients primarily managed for either alcoholic liver cirrhosis or chronic pancreatitis.

Conclusions: Significant common alcoholic damage of liver and pancreas is surprisingly uncommon. This phenomenon is difficult to explain and the answer could be associated with different pathogenesis of particularly alcoholic organ damage.

112

Clinical Features and Management of Focal Pancreatic Lesions in Patients with Normal Remaining Parenchyma

T. Hucl[1], *M. Benes*[1], *J. Fronek*[2], *V. Kral*[3], *P. Pafko*[4], *J. Leffler*[5], *M. Ryska*[2], *J. Spicak*[1]

[1]Dept. of Hepatogastroenterology, [2]Dept. of Surgery, Institute for Clinical and Experimental Medicine, Prague; [3]Dept. of Surgery I, University Hospital, Olomouc; [4]Dept. of Surgery III, [5]Dept. of Surgery I, University Hospital Motol, Prague, Czech Republic

Background: Despite all the advances in imaging methods it remains to be difficult to clearly differentiate between chronic pancreatitis (CP) and pancreatic carcinoma (PC) in patients with a focal pancreatic lesion.

Aims and Methods: We retrospectively analyzed clinical features and management of 94 patients consecutively diagnosed in our departments with a focal pancreatic lesion demonstrated on CT, US or EUS and normal remaining parenchyma.

Results: A total of 94 patients with focal pancreatic lesions were enrolled. A correct final diagnosis was established by histology and clinical follow-up. The patients with CP (11, 11.7%) were predominantly younger (mean age 54.2 years, range 30–71), male and presenting with pain. In comparison, the patients with PC (83, 88.3%) were rather older (mean age 63.7 years, range 36–82), with equal sex distribution and presenting with dyspepsia, pain and jaundice. The most common ERCP finding in focal lesions of the head of the pancreas was stenosis of bile and pancreatic ducts in both conditions. Serum tumor marker CA19-9 was elevated in 18.2% of patients with CP and 75% with PC. Cytology obtained from FNA showed malignant cells in none of the CP patients and in 59.3% of patients with PC. All patients with CP were treated by pancreatic head or tail resection whereas in the group of PC resection was carried out only in 26.2%.

Conclusion: Focal chronic pancreatitis is associated with similar clinical and morphological features that are found in pancreatic carcinoma. Thus, clearly distinguishing benign focal CP from malignant PC remains to be challenging.

113

Pancreatic Fistula following Pancreatic Head Resection for Chronic Pancreatitis – An Impact of the Procedure?

W. Schlosser, D. Henne-Bruns

Department of Visceral- and Transplant Surgery, University of Ulm, Germany

Introduction: The morbidity following pancreatic resection could be reduced significantly during the last decade. However, the morbidity rate is even in specialized centers between 40–60%. The leakage of the pancreatic anastomosis is still the most severe complication in this type of operation. We report of our experience with the management of these complications.

Methods and patients: 456 patients with chronic pancreatitis, who were operated between January 1990 and April 2004 with a pancreatic head resection, were analyzed prospectively. The patients were divided into two groups according to their operative procedure: pylorus-preserving pancreaticoduodenectomy (PPPD; n = 107 patients) and duodenum-preserving pancreatic head resection (DPPHR; n = 349 patients). Prior to surgery the patients had a median medical treatment of 41 month (PPPD) and 45 month (DPPHR), respectively.

Results: Hospital mortality was 0.4% (PPPD 0.9%; DPPHR 0.3%). The morbidity following PPPD was 35% compared to 20% after DPPHR. Local complications were more frequent after PPPD (26%) compared to DPPHR (15%); however, the frequency of pancreatic leakage was similar for both procedures with 5% and 4%, respectively. 7% of the patients operated with PPPD suffered from delayed gastric emptying in the postoperative course. There was no difference in the occurrence of systemic complications (PPPD 8%, DPPHR 5%). Reoperations were necessary in 6% of the patients, mainly due to bleeding or septic complications. The median hospitalization was 15 days (PPPD) and 14 days, respectively.

Conclusion: The mortality for the resection of the pancreatic head for chronic pancreatitis is less than 1% in experienced institutions. The frequency of surgical complications are similar for PPPD and DPPHR, whereas PPPD is associated with a significantly higher incidence of delayed gastric emptying. The leakage of the pancreatic anastomosis is similar for both procedures. Today, pancreatic fistulas can be managed by drainage in most cases and reoperation is only necessary in few patients.

114

Interventional Endoscopy is not Effective for Pain Relief in Patients with Chronic Pancretitis and Main Pancreatic Duct Obstruction

S. Kahl[1], *K. Schuette*[1], *K. Moenkemueller*[1], *H.-U. Schulz*[2], *P. Malfertheiner*[1]

[1]Department of Gastroenterology, Hepatology and Infectious Diseases, [2]Department of Surgery, Otto-von-Guericke-University of Magdeburg, Germany

Introduction: Pancreatic ductal hypertension is described to be associated with pain in chronic pancreatitis (CP). To evaluate pain scores and use of analgesics in patients with CP prior and after interventional endoscopy for prepapillary main pancreatic duct (MPD) strictures. To evaluate characteristics to predict failure or success of interventional endoscopy.

Methods: 39 patients (mean age 44 years, 31 male) underwent interventional endoscopy with sphincterotomy and dilatation of the stricture of the MPD, and stenting with 7- and 10 Fr-Stents for a one year period. Pain scores were measured prior and during interventional endoscopy and after stent removal. Type and amount of used analgesics were reported.

Results: Pain scores prior [median 4 (max 7, min 2)], during [4 (max 7, min 1)] and after [4 (max 8, min 1)] interventional endoscopy were not statistically significant different. Type and amount of necessary analgesics did not change during and after interventional endoscopy, compared to baseline. In 10 patients pain scores increased, in 14 patients pain scores decreased after endoscopic intervention, without any statistical significance. In both groups we could not identify any characteristics (gender, age, endocrine and exocrine insufficiency, enlarged pancreatic head, continued alcohol abuse, duration of CP) to predict outcome of interventional endoscopy. At 29 months follow up only 7 patients (29.2%) had decreased pain scores compared to baseline levels. But even this scores were statistically not significant different.

Conclusions: Compared to reported data in the literature we found interventional endoscopy to be less effective in pain relief in patients with CP. Based on these findings pain in patients with CP is unlikely to be related to ductal obstruction of the MPD. Therefore interventional endoscopy is not the method of choice to treat pain in these patients.

Clinical Pancreatic Cancer

115

PET/CT Influence on Clinical Management of Patients with Pancreatic Neoplasms

C. Sperti[1], C. Pasquali[1], S. Bissoli[2], V. Fiore[2], F. Chierichetti[2], G. Liessi[3], S. Pedrazzoli[1]

[1]Departments of Medical and Surgical Sciences, University of Padua; Departments of [2]Nuclear Medicine, and [3]Radiology, Castelfranco Hospital, Castelfranco Veneto, Treviso, Italy

Introduction: Differential diagnosis of pancreatic masses remains difficult despite the introduction of several technologies. The integrated PET/CT scanner provides the advantage of image fusion in the same examination, improving the anatomic delineation of PET. The aim of this study was to assess the impact of PET/CT on the management of patients with suspected pancreatic tumours.

Methods: From January 2004 to November 2004, 75 patients underwent PET/CT examination for diagnosis and staging of suspected pancreatic neoplasm (n = 53) or during the follow-up after resection for pancreatic cancer (n = 22). CA 19-9 assay and abdominal ultrasonography was also performed. All PET/CT findings were confirmed by operation, biopsy or follow-up.

Results: Thirty-one males and 44 females (mean age of 61.1 years, range 37–80) were included. Twenty-five patients had malignant tumours (24 adenocarcinomas, 1 lymphoma) and 28 a benign disease (12 serous cystadenomas. 8 chronic pancreatitis, 6 IPMN, 2 undefined). PET was positive in 26 pancreatic lesions (25 malignant, p.p.v. 96%); none of the PET negative patients had cancer (n.p.v.: 100%). PET/CT detected distant metastases in 10 patients, 6/10 not seen by conventional imaging, and correctly identified as malignant 6 lesions with inconclusive findings on traditional imaging. Two patients required additional colic resection for simultaneous colon cancer not seen by conventional staging. Recurrent disease occurred in 8 out of 22 patients studied in the follow-up after resection of primary tumour; four were identified only by PET/CT. In one additional patient PET/CT detected a second primary colon carcinoma. Overall, the management was changed in 15 patients (20%).

Conclusions: The management of patients with suspected primary or recurrent pancreatic cancer was changed in 1/5 of patients. We suggest the use of PET/CT in the preoperative work-up of pancreatic neoplasms and in the follow-up after resection of pancreatic adenocarcinoma.

116

Pre- and Postoperative Immunotherapy with Interleukin-2 Enhances Eosinophil Blood Cells in Pancreatic Cancer Patients

C. Nobili, L. Degrate, E. Perego, C. Franciosi, Fr. Uggeri

Department of Surgery, San Gerardo Hospital, University of Milano-Bicocca, Monza (Milano), Italy

Introduction: Recent evidences indicate a crucial role of eosinophils in tumor eradication through the secretion of several molecules, which promote tumor cells destruction and trigger an efficient CD4- and CD8-dependent anticancer immune response. In patients with solid malignancies interleukin-2 immunotherapy is known to induce marked eosinophilia, resulting in a better prognosis. We assessed the effect of pre- and postoperative administration of recombinant IL-2 (rIL-2) on eosinophil blood cells in patients with pancreatic cancer.

Methods: 12 patients with resectable pancreatic adenocarcinoma (8 males, 4 females, mean age = 65 years) received immunotherapy with rIL-2, consisting in a preoperative subcutaneous administration of 12 millions IU/day for 3 consecutive days and a postoperative cycle (on 30th day) of 3 millions IU/day for 6 consecutive days. Percentage and absolute number of eosinophils in peripheral blood were evaluated before administration of rIL-2, on 7th, 14th, 30th postoperative days and 1 month later the postoperative rIL-2 cycle (60th day).

Results: After preoperative rIL-2 administration and radical surgery, the eosinophils percentage and number significantly increased on 7th postoperative day compared with basal values (6.3 ± 3.3% vs. 2.7 ± 1.7%, p = 0,004; 844 ± 588/mmc vs. 183 ± 128/mmc, p = 0.001). In the following period we observed a decline of eosinophils, although they remained constantly and significantly higher than basal levels, reaching values of 6.2 ± 3.3% and 422 ± 302/mmc on 60th day, 1 month after the postoperative rIL-2 cycle (p = 0.01).

Conclusions: These results confirm the rIL-2 action on eosinophil blood cells in a group of pancreatic cancer patients. The elevation of eosinophils percentage and number obtained with a pre- and postoperative rIL-2 immunotherapy is statistically significant and it lasts till 60 days after surgery. The high levels of eosinophils can help immuno-surveillance against the minimal residual disease and they may improve the overall survival of pancreatic cancer patients.

117

Role of Preoperative High Dose Interleukin-2 Immunotherapy in Rising Natural Killer Cells Count in Operable Pancreatic Cancer Patients

L. Degrate, E. Perego, C. Nobili, C. Franciosi, Fa. Uggeri, Fr. Uggeri

Department of Surgery, San Gerardo Hospital, University of Milano-Bicocca, Monza (Milano), Italy

Introduction: An important role in host anticancer defense is played by natural killer (NK) cells, lymphocytes exhibiting natural cytotoxicity against a broad range of tumors. Cancer patients with high levels of NK cells in peripheral blood show a lower incidence of metastases and a better prognosis. Major surgery impairs natural cytotoxicity, promoting the dissemination of tumor cells in the perioperative period. Interleukin-2 is a cytokine able to stimulate the innate immunity against cancer cells, by expanding the number of circulating NK cells and activating their cytotoxic activity. This study was conducted to investigate the influence of preoperative administration of high doses recombinant IL-2 (rIL-2) on blood NK cells in patients with pancreatic adenocarcinoma.

Methods: Twelve consecutive patients with resectable pancreatic adenocarcinoma (8 males, 4 females, mean age = 65 years) underwent subcutaneous immunotherapy with high dose rIL-2 (6 million IU twice a day) for 3 consecutive days prior to surgical radical resection (R0). We measured NK cells level in peripheral blood before rIL-2 administration and on 7th, 14th, 30th post-operative days. Ten patients underwent pancreaticoduodenectomy, 1 splenopancreatectomy and 1 total pancreatectomy.

Results: The toxicity profile was moderate (grade 1–2 of WHO criteria). NK cells in the basal evaluation were 215 ± 117/mmc, while in the post-operative period, comparing to basal values, their number significantly increased to 347 ± 120/mmc ($p = 0.008$) on 7th day, 294 ± 52/mmc ($p = 0.05$) on 14th and 318 ± 135/mmc ($p = 0.03$) on 30th day.

Conclusions: The results of this preliminary work, conducted on patients affected by pancreatic adenocarcinoma, demonstrate that preoperative high dose (12 million IU/day) rIL-2 administration is able to counteract surgery-induced deficiency of NK cells. Considering the important role of NK cells in anticancer defense, the immunotherapy-induced rising of their blood count may be associated with a prolonged survival of pancreatic cancer patients.

118

Clinical Significance of Interleukin-1β and Interleukin-6 Gene Polymorphisms in Pancreatic Adenocarcinoma and Chronic Pancreatitis

R. Talar-Wojnarowska[1], A. Gasiorowska[1], B. Smolarz[2], H. Romanowicz-Makowska[2], J. Strzelczyk[3], A. Janiak[4], E. Malecka-Panas[1]

[1]Department of Digestive Tract Diseases, Medical University of Lodz, [2]Laboratory of Molecular Genetics, Institute of Polish Mother's Memorial Hospital, Lodz, [3]Department of Transplantology, Medical University of Lodz, [4]Department of Gastrointestinal Surgery, Medical University of Lodz, Poland

Background: Many pro-inflammatory cytokines, including interleukin-1 (IL-1) and interleukin-6 (IL-6), contribute to the cachexia associated with pancreatic adenocarcinoma (PA) and may be related to shortened survival time in PA patients. The clinical significance of G-174C IL-6 and *TaqI* IL-1β polymorphisms in pancreatic adenocarcinoma and chronic pancreatitis (CP) has been investigated.

Methods: The study included 49 patients operated for pancreatic adenocarcinoma (26 subjects, 10 men and 16 women) or chronic pancreatitis (23 subjects, 14 men and 9 women). G-174C IL-6 and *TaqI* IL-1β polymorphisms have been studied in genomic DNA isolated from pancreatic tissue after operation. Survival probabilities in patients with PA were computed using univariate Kaplan-Meier analysis.

Results: The genotype frequencies of IL-1β and IL-6 polymorphisms were similar in patients with pancreatic adenocarcinoma and chronic pancreatitis ($p > 0.5$). In PA patients, the correlation between presence of homozygous −174G/G IL-6 genotype and tumor size > 3 cm has been found. Moreover, a significant relationship between the type of IL-6 polymorphism and survival time has been observed. The presence of at least one C allele at position −174 was associated with longer survival of PA patients (11.2 months compared with 4.5 months in GG homozygous; $p < 0.01$). In contrast, the *TaqI* IL-1β polymorphism was not associated with any clinical data.

Conclusion: These results support the hypothesis that polymorphism of IL-6 may play an important role in clinical outcome of pancreatic adenocarcinoma and homozygous −174 G/G may be associated with unfavourable prognosis of this disease.

Work supported by Medical University of Lodz, grant 502-11-042.

119

Development of a Method to Obtain Pancreatic Tissue Samples by Endoscopic Ultrasound (EUS)-Guided Fine Needle Aspiration (FNA)

J. Iglesias-García[1], A. Lozano-Leon[1], J. Lariño-Noia[1], I. Abdulkader[2], J. Antunez[2], J. Forteza[2], J.E. Domínguez-Muñoz[1]

[1]Departments of Gastroenterology and [2]Pathology, University Hospital of Santiago de Compostela, Spain

Introduction: EUS-guided FNA has improved the diagnostic approach to pancreatic lesions. Nevertheless, the efficacy of the method is limited by the obtention of material for cytological study. We develop a method process FNA samples to obtain a core specimen for histological study. The impact of this new method on the diagnostic efficacy of EUS guided FNA is evaluated.

Patients and Methods: 34 consecutive patients (mean age 59 years, range 47–74, 19 male) were prospectively included in the study. EUS was performed under conscious sedation by the lineal scanning Pentax FG-38UX echoendoscope. Punction was made by a 22G needle (Sonotip II, Mediglobe®). In all cases a minimum of three passes were made. In the first pass the sample was processed for cytological study by expelling the sample on a microscope slide using air and the needle stylet. In the second and third passes, tissue samples for histological evaluation were obtained by expelling the core specimen with saline solution from the needle into formol 10%. Results are shown as median and standard deviation. Diagnostic sensitivity is shown in percentage.

Results: Tissue samples for histological study were obtained in all cases (100%). The length of the core specimen was 0.65 ± 0.53 cm (range 0.1–2.2 cm). Diagnosis was reached in 17 patients (50%) by cytology and in 28 patients (82%) by histology. Thus, the histological study increased diagnostic sensitivity of pancreatic FNA by 32%. There were one complication (acute pancreatitis) related with the technique (morbidity 2.9%), without mortality.

Conclusions: Expelling of pancreatic tissue samples after EUS-FNA by injection of saline solution through the needle into formol allows obtaining core specimens for histological study in all cases. This technique leads to a significant improvement in the diagnostic sensitivity of EUS-FNA.

120

Survival Analysis according to Treatment Modality in Pancreatic Cancer Patients

C.D. Kim, S.W. Jung, Y.S. Kim, H.S. Lee, H.J. Chun, S.H. Um, J.H. Hyun

Department of Internal Medicine, Institute of Digestive Disease and Nutrition, Korea University College of Medicine, Seoul, Korea

Introduction: Pancreatic cancer is the 6th leading cause of cancer death in Korea and its incidence is increasing. At present, surgical resection offers the best chance of cure. However, most of pancreatic cancers are already unresectable at diagnosis. Thus, the majority of patients depend on chemotherapy, radiation therapy, or supportive care. We investigated the effect of treatment modalities on the survival in pancreatic cancer.

Methods: Between September 1994 and May 2003, 154 patients with pancreatic cancer were treated by surgery, radiotherapy, chemotherapy and conservative management. The data was analyzed retrospectively for survival according to stage and treatment modality.

Results: Median survival time of patients was 5.7 months and 1 year survival rate was 18.3%. In patients with stage I to III disease, the median survival time was 13.9 months in surgery group, 10.2 months in radiation therapy group, and 6.1 months in supportive care group ($p < 0.01$). Survival rate according to treatment modality was significantly different in this group. In patients with stage IV disease, the median survival time was 6.1 months in radiation therapy group, 7.1 months in chemotherapy group, and 2.7 months in supportive care group. Overall survival was significantly higher in treatment groups than in supportive care group ($p < 0.01$), but there was no difference in survival between chemotherapy group and radiation therapy group.

Conclusions: In patients with stage I to III disease, surgery can improve median survival and in patients with stage IV, either chemotherapy or radiotherapy can prolong survival compared to supportive care. These results suggest that more active treatment of pancreatic cancer even in advanced stage will be needed to prolong survival.

121

Plasma Tumour-M2-Pyruvate Kinase (Tu-M2-PK) and Serum Carbohydrate Antigen (CA 19-9) for the Pre-Operative Diagnosis of Pancreatic Cancer

H.P.P. Siriwardana[1], N.K.K. King[1], M.W. France[2], A.K. Siriwardena[1]

[1]Hepatobiliary Unit and [2]Department of Clinical Biochemistry, Manchester Royal Infirmary, Manchester, UK

Introduction: Many human tumours express pyruvate kinase and an enzyme-linked immunosorbent assay (ELISA) allows reliable detection of tumour-M2-pyruvate kinase (Tu-M2-PK) in blood. This study assesses the value of Tu-M2-PK, either alone or in conjunction with carbohdyrate antigen (CA 19-9) for the pre-operative diagnosis of peri-ampullary cancer.

Methods: 104 consecutive patients with suspected peri-ampullary cancer underwent venesection with informed consent. 77 (74%) had subsequent histological confirmation of peri-ampullary malignancy and constitute the study population. Median age (range) was 68 (26–82) years and 46 were jaundiced at sampling. Controls were patients undergoing cholecystectomy (with normal liver function) and jaundiced patients without evidence of malignancy at ERCP. CA 19-9 and Tu-M2-PK were assayed prior to resection or biopsy. Principal outcomes were sensitivity and specificity of Tu-M2-PK and CA 19-9 individually and in combination for diagnosis of peri-ampullary cancer.

Results: Mean (standard error) plasma Tu-M2-PK in patients with malignancy was 41.2 (26.7) U/ml and for controls was 29.1 (21.3) U/ml (Mann-Whitney U, $p = 0.004$). Tu-M2-PK was unaffected by serum bilirubin (Spearman rho = 0.148, $p = 0.084$). Using Receiver operator curves, optimal cut-off for differentiating controls from patients with histologically confirmed malignancy for Tu-M2-PK was 27 U/ml and 38.5 U/ml for CA 19-9. The area under the curve was 0.669 for Tu-M2-PK, 0.833 for CA 19-9 and 0.842 for Tu-M2-PK + CA 19-9 ($p < 0.01$) combined.

Conclusions: The combination of Tu-M2-PK and CA 19-9 appears more effective than either test used in isolation and can augment imaging and cytologic information for the pre-operative diagnosis of peri-ampullary cancer.

122

Antecolic Reconstruction Reduces Delayed Gastric Emptying following Pylorus-Preserving Pancreaticoduodenectomy

M.N. Wente[1], M. Hartel[1], U. Hinz[1], J. Kleeff[1], M. Wagner[2], M.W. Müller[1], H. Friess[1], M.W. Büchler[1]

[1]Department of General Surgery, University of Heidelberg, Germany; [2]Department of Visceral and Transplantation Surgery, University of Berne, Switzerland

Introduction: A major complication following pancreatic surgery is delayed gastric emptying (DGE). The influence of antecolic or retrocolic reconstruction of the duodenojejunostomy on DGE following pylorus-preserving pancreaticoduodenectomy (ppW) remains unclear.

Methods: The experience with antecolic or retrocolic duodenojejunostomy in ppW has been analyzed using a prospective database and univariate and multivariate models. 100 consecutive patients undergoing ppW with retrocolic reconstruction between 1996 and 2001, and 100 consecutive patients undergoing ppW with antecolic reconstruction between 2002 and 2003 were evaluated. Characteristics like median age, median hospital stay, gender, diagnosis, prior operations, blood loss, surgical and medical complications, ASA risk groups, stent implantation and especially DGE were matched for the comparison groups.

Results: DGE occurred significantly more in patients with retrocolic reconstruction than in patients with antecolic reconstruction ($p < 0.001$). The ante- and retrocolic study groups were comparable regarding patient age ($p = 0.248$), gender ($p = 0.48$), postoperative surgical and medical complications ($p = 0.19$, and $p = 0.054$, respectively). The univariate analysis between patients with and without DGE did not show significant differences regarding diagnosis, prior operations, blood loss, surgical and medical complications, ASA classification, or stent implantation. In the multivariate analysis only the way of reconstruction ($p = 0.006$) and gender ($p = 0.04$) seems to influence DGE.

Conclusions: Antecolic duodenojejunostomy in patients undergoing pylorus-preserving pancreaticoduodenectomy (ppW) seems to be the favorable approach to reduce the risk of delayed gastric emptying.

123

Neural Sprouting and Neural Hypertrophy in Pancreatic Ductal Adenocarcinoma is Related to the High Expressions of GAP-43, NGF and Artemin

G.O. Ceyhan[1], A.G. Kerscher[1], F. Bergmann[2], M. Müller[1], N.Giese[1], M. Erkan[1], T. Giese[3], M.W. Büchler[1], H. Friess[1]

[1]Department of General Surgery, [2]Institute of Pathology, [3]Institute for Immunology, University of Heidelberg, Germany

Introduction: Pancreatic-ductal-adeno-carcinoma (PDAC) is characterized by local nerve alterations and perineural invasion. Neural sprouting and hypertrophy of intra-pancreatic nerves were analyzed in PDAC with correlation to the neurotrophic factors; GAP-43, NGF and artemin.

Methods: Intrapancreatic nerves in tissue sections of normal pancreas (NP) ($n = 45$), histologically normal pancreas next to pancreatic cancer (NNPC) ($n = 48$) and in PDAC ($n = 52$) were immunostained using the pan-neuronal marker PGP9.5. Quantification of the nerve number and nerve cross-section area were made by using the Zeiss KS300 program. Expressions of GAP-43, NGF, and artemin were investigated by immunohistochemistry, QRT-PCR and Western blot analysis.

Results: Quantitative analysis of intrapancreatic nerves revealed a significant increase in neural sprouting in NNPC ($p < 0.0001$) and PDAC ($p < 0.001$) compared to NP. Furthermore the cross-sectional area of nerves in NNPC ($p < 0.0002$) and PDAC ($p < 0.00000005$) was much bigger compared to NP as it was also significantly bigger in PDAC ($p < 0.0005$) compared to NNPC. Although the GAP-43 immunoreactivity was generally absent in NP, in NNPC and PDAC strong staining in all nerves, especially in the hypertrophic ones was detected. These findings were confirmed by Western blot and QRT-PCR analysis in terms of protein and RNA expression of GAP-43. Similar results were also obtained in the expression analyses of NGF and Artemin. Regarding only PDAC, GAP-43 protein expression was directly correlated to enlarged neural hypertrophy, whereas NGF protein accumulation was mostly seen in mild intrapancreatic neural hypertrophy.

Conclusions: PDAC is associated with increased neural sprouting and neural hypertrophy. Neural hypertrophy is also present in histologically normal areas next to pancreatic cancer and further increases in areas of cancer. These changes of intrapancreatic nerves are directly related to the significantly increased levels of the neurotrophic factors GAP-43, NGF and Artemin in PDAC.

124

Contribution of Peripheral Blood Mononuclear Cells to Cachexia in Patients Suffering from Pancreatic Cancer

M.E. Martignoni, P. Kunze, N. Giese, J. Bachmann, B. Fröhlich, M.W. Büchler, H. Friess

Department of General Surgery, University of Heidelberg, Germany

Introduction: The development of cachexia is a substantial prognostic step in patients suffering from various cancers. The reasons for the development of tumor-cachexia are still not fully clarified. In preliminary studies the co-culture between PBMCs and pancreatic cancer cells as a model of the interaction between tumor-cells and immuncompetent cells of the patient has been established. It was now the aim of this study to clarify which pathomechanisms in cachexia are mediated via PBMCs.

Methods: In 16 Patients with pancreatic cancer (7 Pat. with / 9 Pat. without cachexia) and in 9 controls a co-culture with 2 pancreatic cancer cell-lines (T3M4&Panc-1) and isolated PBMCs was implemented. The cells have no physical contact between each other and are only able to communicate via the cell medium. Thereafter the production of IL-8, IL-1β, TNF-α and UCP-2 of the PBMCs was analysed by RQT-PCR.

Results: In PBMCs of all three groups co-cultured with the IL-6 negative tumor cell-line Panc-1 only an unspecific increase of IL-8 and Il-1β mRNA expression was observed. In contrast, PBMCs of patients with pancreatic cancer and cachexia revealed a significant increase (up to 10x) in the expression of IL-8 and IL-1β when co-cultured with the cytokine-positive cell-line T3M4. However, there was no change in mRNA expression of TNF-α and UCP-2 in the PBMCs of these patients.

Conclusion: PBMCs of pancreatic cancer patients with cachexia can be triggered by tumor-cells to produce cachexia inducing cytokines like IL-8 and IL-1β. However, not all cytokines involved in cachexia are mediated via this mechanism. UCP-2 and TNF-α which play an important role in the profuse muscle degradation are up-regulated via a different pathomechanism. This shows that an interaction of host derived cytokines and expression of cachexia inducing cytokines released by the tumor may be a critical step in the development of cancer cachexia.

125

The Role of the Portal-Mesenteric Vein Resection for the Pancreatic Head Carcinoma

T. Hatori[1], A. Fukuda[1], S. Onizawa[1], N. Kanai[1], T. Oohara[1], T. Imaizumi[2], K. Takasaki[1]

[1]Department of Gastroenterological Surgery, Tokyo Women's Medical University, Tokyo, Japan, [2]Department of Gastroenterological Surgery, School of Medicine, Tokai University, Isehara, Japan

Background: The pancreatic head carcinoma often infiltrates to the portal-mesenteric vein and extrapancreatic nerve plexuses easily because of the anatomical relationship between pancreatic head and portal-mesenteric vein. Therefore, the portal-mesenteric vein resection is sometimes required to remove the tumor completely in case that the tumor invasion to the portal-mesenteric vein is suspicious or obvious.

Objective: The aim of this study is to clarify the role of the portal-mesenteric vein resection for the pancreatic head carcinoma.

Methods: A total of 452 patients who underwent radical operation for the pancreatic head carcinoma without distant metastases between 1978 and 2003 were chosen in this study. 270 patients who underwent portal-mesenteric vein resection (PVR+) were compared with 182 patients who didn't undergo portal-mesenteric vein resection (PVR–). In PVR+, 175 patients (65%) had positive invasion of the portal-mesenteric vein, histopathologically.

Results: There were no differences in background characteristics between the groups, including age, gender, mortality and morbidity. However, the advanced stage rates were seen higher in PVR+ than in PVR–. The 5-year survival rates were 9% in PVR+, 21% in PVR–. In the patients without tumor invasion to the portal-mesenteric vein, R0 rates were 59% in PVR+, 66% in PVR–. The 5-year survival rates were 25% in PVR+ with R0, 0% in PVR+ with R1, 31% in PVR– with R0, 6% in PVR– with R1, respectively. There were no differences between the groups. However, the rate of the tumor invasion to the extrapancreatic nerve plexuses in PVR+ was higher with 52% than 38% in PVR– ($p < 0.05$). In the patients with tumor invasion to the portal-mesenteric vein, all patients underwent PVR and R0 rate was 40%. The 5-year survival rates were 14% in R0 patients, 3% in R1 patients ($p < 0.05$).

Conclusion: It was suggested that the portal-mesenteric vein resection could help dissection of the extrapancreatic nerve plexuses in the pancreatic head carcinoma and lead R0 resection.

126

Pancreatic Fistula is Preceded by Post-Operative Subclinical Pancreatitis after Pancreatic Resection

S. Räty, J. Sand, I. Nordback

Department of Gastroenterology and Alimentary Tract Surgery, Tampere University Hospital, Finland

Background: Pancreatic fistula is the most common complication after pancreatic resection. 'Soft pancreas' is more vulnerable to fistula development, but the pathophysiology of this complication is far from clear. In this study we analyzed pancreatic changes by serial urine trypsinogen strip-test (U-TT) and CT scan in relation to fistula formation.

Patients and Methods: 50 consecutive patients undergoing pancreatic resection (38 PPPD, 5 Whipple's, 5 body/tail resections, 1 Beger, 1 enucleation), were included. There were 28 males, 22 females, median age 65 (7–84) yrs. There were 25 ductal adenocarcinomas, 3 bile duct carcinomas, 1 duodenal carcinoma, 2 carcinoid tumours, 1 endocrine carcinoma, 2 IPMTs, 2 mucinous tumours, 3 insulinomas, 1 bile duct adenoma, 1 serous cystadenoma and 9 chronic pancreatitis. Drain output and amylase activity were measured on post-operative day 4 and 6 (fistula: > 50 ml of fluid with amylase 3 times over normal serum rate), CT scan on day 2 and 6 and U-TT (Actim Pancreatitis®) daily on day 1–7.

Results: 12 patients (24%) developed pancreatic fistula, 11 being subclinical and 1 requiring re-operation. The patients with fistula had often preceding pancreatitis according to CT scan (9/12 vs. 3/38, p = 0.001). Sensitivity and specificity of U-TT to predict CT diagnosed pancreatitis was 100% and 89% and fistula formation 92% and 87%.

Conclusions: Post-operative pancreatic fistula after pancreatic resection is associated with post-operative pancreatitis that can be reliably diagnosed early by urine trypsinogen strip-test.

127

Frequency of K-ras Mutations in Fine Needle Aspiration (FNA) Samples of Pancreatic Adenocarcinoma

C. Šálek[1,2], L. Benešová[2], M. Jelínková[2], P. Hrabal[3], M. Zavoral[1], M. Minárik[2]

[1]Department of Gastroenterology, Institute for Postgraduate Medical Education; [2]Laboratory for Molecular Oncology, Genomac International; [3]Department of Pathology, Central Military Hospital, Prague, Czech Republic

Background: Activation of K-ras oncogene by somatic point mutations is an early event in pancreatic cancerogenesis. It is found in premalignant lesions with frequency about 40% in PanIN 1 and 80% in PanIN 2. Occurrence of K-ras mutations reaches up to 90% in developed pancreatic cancer (PC). Monitoring of K-ras status is considered as a potential tool in early detection of PC. Numerous groups have demonstrated detection of K-ras mutations in PC resection tissues, pancreatic duct brushings, percutaneous biopsies and plasma; this is the report on sensitive detection of K-ras mutations directly in FNA biopsy tissue.

Methods: FNA biopsies were taken from a total of 35 individuals diagnosed with suspicious pancreatic mass during endoscopic ultrasonography. The aspirates were evaluated cytologically and were subjected to molecular-genetic analysis of K-ras mutations. The definite malignant status of the tumors was confirmed from resections following a surgery and/or a long-term follow-up.

Results: Of 30 patients with confirmed PC status, 21 (70%) exhibited malignant positivity for both, cytology and K-ras test, 2 patients (6.7%) had negative cytology test while carrying a K-ras mutation and 3 patients (10%) had positive cytology with no K-ras mutations. In 4 patients (13.3%) with subsequently confirmed PC neither of the two tests was positive. All detected K-ras mutations were located in codon 12 of exon 1. Sensitivity of single cytologic evaluation was 80%, that of cytology combined with K-ras test reached 90%.

Conclusions: The results confirmed high frequency of K-ras mutations in bioptic tissue samples from PC. FNA biopsy was approved as a suitable method of sampling for molecular diagnostics. Tumor targeted approach in which genetic alterations are detected directly from cancerous cells collected from cytology smears should increase the sensitivity of the K-ras testing, and open a possibility to include other molecular markers such as p16, DPC4 and p53.

128

Performances of k-*ras* Oncogene Mutation Analysis in Cytological Material Sampled by EUS-Guided Fine Needle Aspiration for the Diagnosis of Pancreatic Cancer

M. Bouisson[1], B. Bournet[1], P. Hammel[2], A. Aubert[2], P. Lévy[2], P. Ruszniewski[2], N. Vaysse[1], J. Escourrou[1], L. Buscail[1]

[1]Department of Gastroenterology and INSERM U531, CHU Rangueil, Toulouse; [2]Department of Gastroenterology, Hôpital Beaujon, Clichy, France

Introduction: Mutation of k-*ras* oncogene is found in 80 to 90% of pancreatic carcinoma (PC) tissues. Performances of k-*ras* mutation analysis in pancreatic juice sampled during ERCP were: sensitivity 67%, specificity 85% with a failure of DNA amplification in 13% of cases (Berthelémy et al. Ann Int Med 1995; Costentin et al. Pancreatology 2002). Accuracy of EUS-guided fine needle aspiration/biopsy (EUS-FNA) for diagnosis of solid tumor range from 74 to 85%. Aim of the study was to determine the performances of k-*ras* mutation analysis in the cytological material sampled by EUS-FNA for the diagnosis of PC.

Patients and Methods: EUS-FNA samples from 59 pancreatic solid tumors (59 patients, M: 42, W: 17, mean age 60 years, 32–85 yrs) were analysed for k-*ras* mutation using DNA extraction/RFLP following by direct sequencing in case of positive result. Analysis was made retrospectively when final diagnosis have been obtained: adenocarcinoma n = 41, chronic pancreatitis n = 8 and other lesions n = 10 (endocrine tumor, metastasis, other tumors).

Results: DNA amplification failed in only 2 cases (3.4%). k-*ras* mutation was found in 32 cases of adenocarcinoma, 1 case of chronic pancreatitis and 1 case of endocrine carcinoma. Diagnosis values for pancreatic cancer were finally including failure of DNA amplification: sensitivity 78%, specificity 89%, accuracy 79.5%.

Conclusion: According to this bi-centric evaluation, diagnosis performances of k-*ras* mutation analysis in the cytological material from EUS-FNA are superior to that previously found in pure pancreatic juice from ERCP. This analysis coupled to cytology/histology could increase the yield of EUS-FNA for diagnosis of solid pancreatic lesions.

129

Diabetes in Patients with Pancreatic Cancer

A. Gasiorowska[1], R. Talar-Wojnarowska[1], A. Janiak[2], E. Malecka-Panas[1]

[1]Department of Digestive Tract Diseases, [2]Department of General Surgery and Transplantology, Medical University of Lodz, Poland

Background: Pancreatic cancer is often associated with diabetes, however its clinical course and complications are not well studied yet. The aim of the study was to analyze the incidence, complications and management in patients with pancreatic cancer and diabetes.

Methods: Between 2001 and 2003 a total of 109 patients (53 (49%) men and 56 (51%) women) with pancreatic cancer have been evaluated. The diagnosis of pancreatic cancer was based on clinical, US, CT and pathology. In 88 (81%) patients the tumor was localized in pancreatic head, and in 21 patients (19%) in body and/or tail. Plasma glucose profile and glycated hemoglobin (HbA1c) have been measured. Retinopathy has been evaluated in all patients with pancreatic cancer and diabetes with fundoscopy.

Results: Diabetes has been diagnosed in 32 (28%) patients with pancreatic cancer. Diabetes was more often observed in men (21) than in women (10) ($p < 0.01$). In 17 (55%) of them diabetes was diagnosed in median less then one year prior to the diagnosis of pancreatic cancer. Diabetes was observed in patients with pancreatic head tumor (27 patients), and in body and/or tail tumor (4 patients). 15 patients have been treated with insulin and median insulin dose was 36 IU/day. 16 patients have been treated with oral drugs (glimepiride, gliclazide). Among patients with pancreatic cancer and diabetes control of blood glucose was poor in 8 (25%) (HbA1c > 8) patients with accompanying hypoglycemic attacks in 4 of them. Diabetic retinopathy was diagnosed in 4 patients with history of diabetes longer then five years.

Conclusion: Diabetes represents a frequent event in pancreatic cancer. However its clinical course is usually mild and complications are rare, the tendency to hypoglycemic events needs to be considered.

130

Promoter Methylation Detected in Pancreatic Juice: Relationship with Cancer, Age and Survival

L. Yan[1], L. Vitone[1], J. Earl[1], N. Howes[1], J. Leslie[1], G. Lancaster[2], J. Evans[3], I. Gilmore[4], H. Smart[4], M. Lombard[4], J.P. Neoptolemos[1], W. Greenhalf[1]

[1]Division of Surgery and Oncology, University of Liverpool, [2]Centre for Medical Statistics and Health Evaluation, University of Liverpool, [3]Department of Radiology, Royal Liverpool University Hospital, [4]Depatment of Gastroenterology, Royal Liverpool University Hospital, Liverpool, UK

Introduction: When pancreatic cancer is identified it is normally too late to treat and patients die within a few months; In cancer, genes that would otherwise prevent tumours are switched off by methylation of the regions that promote expression. Detection of promoter methylation in DNA from pancreatic juice extracted from patients could be a marker of early cancer, but promoter methylation has also been reported to increase with age.

Methods: Pancreatic juice was obtained at ERCP from 44 pancreatic ductal adenocarcinoma (PDAC), 26 chronic pancreatitis and 31 Biliary stone patients. Promoter methylation was quantified using real time methylation-specific PCR. Genes and loci were analysed were: p16; hMLH1, MGMT, MINT2, MINT31 and MINT32.

Results: Only p16 promoter methylation differentiated pancreatic cancer patients from controls Median methylation (IQR) for PDAC, pancreatitis and biliary-stone controls were 20.4% (0.48, 35.8); 0.15% (0.09, 0.25); and 0.20% (0.11, 0.46) respectively ($p < 0.001$ Kruskall-Wallis). In our study younger groups of patients tended to have higher (not lower) levels of p16 promoter methylation (this did not reach significance). MLH1 promoter methylation was higher in patients with biliary stones than patients with pancreatitis or cancer and was significantly higher in older (>60) patients ($p < 0.001$ Kruskall-Wallis). We found no evidence that promoter methylation levels on their own are associated with survival, but there is a significant association between low MGMT promoter methylation (<50%) and K-Ras mutation ($p = 0.01$ Fischer's exact). Only one patient had low MGMT promoter methylation and no K-Ras mutation (the patient was 30 years old at ERCP, had a p53 mutation in juice and despite being inoperable was still alive after 2 years).

Conclusions: p16 promoter methylation is useful in identification of cancer patients, but the other promoters investigated here do not significantly increase discrimination. MGMT promoter methylation in pancreatic juice may be associated with wild-type K-Ras.

131

Sensitivity of Brush Cytology and Biopsy from Pancreas and Biliary Ducts

Á. Pap, G. Elek, T. Gyökeres, E. Schäfer

MÁV Hospital, Departments of Pathology and Gastroenterology, Budapest, Hungary

Aim: Endoscopic intraductal biopsy and brush cytology arc routine methods for diagnosis of strictures encountered during ERCP. The disadvantage of these methods is their modest sensitivity due to the relatively high occurrence of false negative results in malignant cases. The aim of this work is to present the preoperative diagnostic efficacy and analyse the false negativity in the period of two years from 1999 to 2000.

Methods: 113 intraductal cytology and 92 intraductal biopsy were taken from 113 patients at ERCP after endoscopic papillotomy. Cytologic specimens were immediately prefixed with Fixative spray, the biopsies placed in 10% buffered formalin and processed later conventionally. For analysis the inconclusive, law or medium grade dysplasia preoperative diagnoses were considered as benign and results that were suggestive for malignancy and/or high grade dysplasia were included in the malignant category. The definitive diagnoses were established either with histology of surgical resections and autopsy or through clinical follow up. According to the definitive histology the preoperative results were retrospectively classified as true negatives or positives and false negatives or positives. All diagnoses were rescreened by a cytopathologist.

Results: Among 90 evaluated patients no false positive was found, 16 were true negatives and 26 false negative preoperatively. Late on revision of the samples revealed 4 malignant cases among the false negative cytologic brushings, 3 of them were interpretive errors (mostly. severe dysplasias) and one case was a technical error. The number of the sampling errors proved to be 24. Four of them were caused by hypocellular brushings. The sampling-, technical- and interpretive errors distributed as ~84%, 4%, 12%, respectively among the 26 preoperative false negative cases.

Conclusions: Significant reduction in false negative diagnoses can be achieved only by development of strict diagnostic criteria and by producing specimens that arc technically perfect with no sampling error. Reclassification of specimens considering the latest criteria (primary and secondary malignant features and PanINs) resulted in improvement of the diagnostic work.

132

Osteopontin Modifies the Invasiveness of Pancreatic Cancer Cells: Potential Therapeutic and Diagnostic Marker

A. Kolb[1], J. Kleeff[1], A. Guweidhi[1], N. Giese[1], H. Adwan[2], T. Giese[1], M.R. Berger[2], M.W. Büchler[1], H. Friess[1]

[1]Department of General Surgery, University of Heidelberg, Germany, [2]Unit of Toxicology and Chemotherapy, German Cancer Research Center (DKFZ), Heidelberg, Germany

Introduction: Pancreatic ductal adenocarcinoma (PDAC) is one of the most aggressive malignancies with an overall 5- year survival rate of less then 5%. Invasive tumor growth and early metastasis are two important reasons for this dismal prognosis. Osteopontin (OPN) is a secretory protein with a variety of functions, in e.g. cell adhesion and migration, inflammatory reaction and apoptosis. OPN can increase tumor growth, invasiveness and metastases, and it has also been suggested to serve as a biological marker in certain tumors.

Methods and Results: In this study the functional role of OPN in human pancreatic cancer and its potential use as a new disease marker were analyzed. By quantitative PCR, there was a 2.5-fold increase of OPN mRNA in pancreatic cancers ($n = 23$) compared to normal pancreatic tissues ($n = 20$) ($p < 0.05$). Immunohistochemical analysis demonstrated OPN staining in 60% of the primary pancreatic tumors and in 72% of the lymphnode and liver metastases. ELISA analysis of serum samples obtained from pancreatic cancer patients ($n = 70$) and healthy donors ($n = 20$) showed a 2.1-fold increase in OPN serum levels in tumor patients. Recombinant human OPN significantly increased the invasiveness of pancreatic cancer cells, without having any impact on cell proliferation. In addition, downregulation of OPN by specific siRNA molecules decreased pancreatic cancer cell invasion.

Conclusions: OPN serum levels in pancreatic cancer patients derive most probably from the increased production of OPN by the tumor cells, thus suggesting a possible role of OPN as a prognostic or follow-up marker. Our results also suggest that blockade of OPN might be useful as a therapeutic approach to inhibit invasion and metastasis of pancreatic cancer cells.

133

Renal Cell Carcinoma Metastatic to the Pancreas

M. Thalhammer[1], S. Altziebler[2], W. Schweiger[1], P. Reittner[3], G. Bernhardt[4], H. Bacher[1], C. Lackner[4], M. Ratschek[4], H.J. Mischinger[1]

Departments of [1]Surgery, [2]Urology, [3]Radiology, [4]Pathology, Medical University of Graz, Austria

Introduction: The diverse natural history of renal cell carcinoma (RCC) includes metastases to the pancreas, a very unusual site for distant spread of other cancers.

Methods: We retrospectively reviewed the records of eleven patients with RCC metastatic to the pancreas, detected by CT examination between 1994 and 2004. All patients had undergone a previous nephrectomy for RCC. The mean interval between resection of the primary RCC and detection of the pancreatic metastases was 74.4 months (range: 0–262.8 months). Surgical resection comprised, 2 Whipple procedures, 7 distal resections and 2 simple enucleations.

Results: In 7 patients (64%) the pancreas was the only site of metastatic disease of RCC. Overall, 8 patients (73%) were alive at a mean of 40.8 months after diagnosis of metastatic disease, 6 of whom without evidence of disease. Two showed local recurrence. Three patients (27%) died, two of metastatic disease, one of postoperative bleeding.

Conclusions: Long-term follow up is very important for patients with RCC, because metastatic disease may be detected decades after the initial diagnosis. The prognosis of RCC metastatic to the pancreas is much better than that for primary pancreatic adenocarcinoma.

134

Usefulness of CT-Guided Splanchnic Nerve Block for Controlling Pancreatic Cancer Pain

A. Fukuda, T. Hatori, S. Onizawa, N. Kanai, T. Ohara, K. Furukawa, K. Takasaki

Department of Surgery, Institute of Gastroenterology, Tokyo Women's Medical University, Tokyo, Japan

Introduction: Efficacy of CT-guided splanchnic nerve block was assessed in 34 patients with unresectable pancreatic cancer or recurrent pancreatic tumor after surgery complaining of sever pain.

Patients and Methods: 34 patients (Mean age:61.0 years old, 17 males and 17 females) had undergone CT-guided splanchnic nerve block since 1997. According to the WHO ladder of the analgesics, 5 patients(15%) had step1, 2 patients (6%) had step2, and 27 patients (79%) had step3 analgesics before the nerve block. Using CT monitor, the needle was inserted from the back into the retrocrural space and the splanchnic neurolysis was performed with alcohol solution (5–60 ml).

Results: Pain was relieved in 29 of 34 patients (85%). The retrocrural space had already been destroyed by the tumor in 4 of 5 patients without pain relief by the nerve block. 8 patients had diarrhea, 4 had hypotension, and 3 had nausea or vomiting. However no severe complication was observed during and after the procedure.

Conclusions: CT-guided splanchnic nerve block was safe and useful for controlling pancreatic cancer pain. However it is desirable to perform it before the destruction of the retrocrural space.

135

The Impact of Cigarette Smoking on Pancreatic Adenocarcinoma Survival, Stage and Location

R.E. Brand[1], A. Nickolov[2], H. Du[2], A. Zisman[1], A. Gorchow[3], R.M. Brand[1]

[1]Department of Medicine, [2]Center on Outcomes, Research and Education, [3]Cancer Registry, Evanston Northwestern Healthcare, Evanston, IL, USA

Introduction: Smoking is the most important environmental risk factor for the development of pancreatic adenocarcinoma (PC). We recently reported that smokers had an earlier age of diagnosis for PC when compared to never smokers (NS) by using data from the IMPAC Medical Registry Services Cancer Information Resource file (CIRF). The CIRF includes data from more than 350 community and teaching hospitals. The aim of this study was to determine the impact of smoking on tumor location, stage at diagnosis and survival by using the CIRF from 1993–2003.

Methods: 29,239 patients diagnosed with a pancreatic cancer consistent with adenocarcinoma were identified. Patients with an unknown cigarette smoking history or cigar/pipe/snuff use were omitted. Survival data was used only on patients from 1993 to 2001 to ensure a minimum 2-year follow-up. Smoking history was classified as NS, current © defined as smoking within 1 year of diagnosis, or previous (P). Cox proportional models, Log-rank test, and Kaplan-Meier survival plots were used.

Results: Smoking status did not effect survival with median survival times of 149 days, 156 days and 148 days for C, P and NS, respectively. Current smokers were more likely to present with a tumor in the tail rather than the head of the pancreas ($p < 0.001$). Stage 3 and 4 tumors were more common for C at 79.4% (odds ratio 1.302, $p < 0.001$) and P at 76.5% (odds ratio 1.095, $p = 0.025$) as compared to NS at 74.8%.

Conclusion: Unlike its effect on age of diagnosis, cigarette smoking does not appear to impact patient survival. This is despite an increase in advanced stage tumors and tail lesions, both of which are adverse prognostic factors. Further studies are needed to better understand why smoking does not appear to influence survival.

136

The Notch Signalling Pathway Determines Neuro-Vascular Progression of Pancreatic Cancer

P. Büchler[1], A. Gazdhar[1], M. Schubert[1], N. Giese[1], H.A. Reber[2], O.J. Hines[2], T. Giese[1], G.O. Ceyhan[1], M. Müller[1], M.W. Büchler[1], H. Friess[1]

[1]Department of General Surgery, University of Heidelberg, Germany; [2]Department of Surgery, UCLA School of Medicine, University of California, Los Angeles, CA, USA

Background: Angiogenesis, pain, and early neuroinvasion are clinical features of pancreatic cancer. Blood vessels and nerves develop together and use common routes through the organism. The Notch pathway (Notch-1/4, Jagged-1/2, Delta) appears crucial in this process. The current study analyzed the Notch pathway in pancreatic cancer and characterized its angiogenic and invasive effects.

Methods: Five PaCa cell lines were cultured for the in vitro experiments. Real-time quantitative RT-PCR was done to quantify mRNA expression in 31 human PaCa specimens, and immunohistochemistry was used to localize protein expression within tumor specimens. Activation of the Notch signalling was done by transfection of PaCa cells with a constitutive active Notch-1 mutant (Notch-IC). Overexpression of Jagged and Delta was achieved by transfection of full-length cDNA. Spheroid assays were utilized to study angiogenesis and ELISAs to measure VEGF, bFGF and angiogenin expression. Matrigel invasion assays were used to analyze tumor cell invasion.

Results: Notch-3 and Notch-4 mRNA were significantly ($p < 0.001$) overexpressed in PaCa. Immunohistochemistry revealed protein accumulation of Notch-1 as well. All ligands were significantly upregulated. A positive immunosignal of ligands was seen in nerves, blood vessels, and ductal tumor cells. Transfection of PaCa cells with the constitutive active Notch-IC mutant and with Jagged-1 revealed increased levels for VEGF. Concomitantly, recombinant Jagged-1 increased sprouting of endothelial cells in the spheroid assay.

Conclusion: The Notch pathway most likely regulates neurovascular development in pancreatic cancer. Activation of this signalling pathway by constitutive Notch-1 mutants and by Jagged-1 causes an angiogenic and invasive tumor phenotype. Specific blockade of Notch signalling may therefore be beneficial for patients with pancreatic cancer.

137

Matriptase – A New Hypoxia Inducible Regulator of Tumor Cell Invasion and Metastasis

P. Büchler[1], Y. Su[1], S. Kelleg[1], M. Schubert[1], N. Giese[1], H.A. Reber[2], O.J. Hines[2], T. Giese[1], M.W. Büchler[1], H. Friess[1]

[1]Department of General Surgery, University of Heidelberg, Germany; [2]Department of Surgery, UCLA School of Medicine, University of California, Los Angeles, CA, USA

Background: A condition of low oxygen is a hallmark in the growth of pancreatic cancer grows and likely induces a specific, yet unknown, gene expression profile. Aim: In the present study we aimed to clone new hypoxia inducible genes and characterize possible new genes in growth of pancreatic cancer.

Methods: Cloning of new hypoxia inducible genes was achieved by the RDA (representative differential analysis) method. Hypoxic induction of identified genes was confirmed by Northern blot analysis and all clones were sequenced. Expression studies in human pancreatic cancer specimens and cell lines were done by real time quantitative PCR and Western blot. Tissue specimens were analyzed by immunohistochemistry and in situ hybridization. Tumor cell invasion was studied with matrigel invasion assays and cell viability with MTT assays. Recombinant overexpression of identified clones was achieved by stable transfection of MIA PaCa-2 cells with the full length cDNA clones.

Results: After hypoxic exposure for 14 h a gene was cloned called, matriptase, in a series of RDA experiments. Hypoxic induction of matriptase expression was confirmed by Northern blot analysis. Analysis of matriptase in pancreatic cancer showed a significant increase of matriptase mRNA and protein levels. Localization of matriptase expression in tissue specimens revealed expression primarily by ductal cancer cells close to the invasion front of tumors. Experimental overexpression of matriptase resulted in an increased invasive tumor phenotype, which was even more pronounced under conditions of low oxygen. Inhibition studies using a specific matriptase inhibitor reverted the invasiveness.

Conclusion: In the present study we have identified matriptase as a new hypoxia inducible gene. Characterization of matriptase gene expression in human tissue specimens and recombinant overexpression of matriptase revealed an important function of this gene in growth of human pancreatic cancer by regulation of tumor cell invasion and metastasis.

138

Oncology Risk Evaluation of Large Pancreatic Cystic Lesions by Endoscopic Ultrasonography Fine Needle Aspiration

A. Pukitis[1], J. Pokrotnieks[1], V. Mikazans[2], A. Skutelis[2]

[1]Gastroenterology Center, Paul Stradinsh Clinical University Hospital, Riga; [2]Latvia Institute of Cardiology, Riga, Latvia

Introduction: Pancreatic cystic lesions bigger than 20 mm have higher suspicion for malignancy. Diagnostic algorithm for the large pancreatic cystic lesions is still on evaluation. Endoscopic ultrasonography guided fine needle aspiration (EUS-FNA) is one of the diagnostic approaches for the pancreatic cystic lesions. Cystic content analysis (cytology, amylase, CEA, CA19-9), for the verification of diagnosis was one the aims of this study.

Methods: In total 25 patients (11 women, 14 men) in an age from 37 to 80 (mean age 58.5 years) with one or more pancreatic cystic lesions (size from 2 to 12 cm) detected by US, EUS, MRI or CT were involved. All pancreatic cystic lesions were examined with EUS-FNA using EUS GF-UC145AL (Olympus®) and ProSound SSD5000 (ALOKA®) technology, NA-10J-1, NA-200H-8022 (Olympus®) and ECHOTIP EUSN-1 (WilsonCook®) standard biopsy needle systems.

Results: EUS showed pancreas parenchyma echodensity changes (n = 16, 63%), cystic lesions with increased risk findings i.e. septae, calcifications, solid structures (n = 9; 37%), pancreatic duct size, structure changes (n = 11; 43%). Surgery treatment was performed in 6 cases (24%). Cytology analysis of the cyst content showed malignant cells (n = 3, 12%), high-grade adenocarcinoma (n = 1), low-grade adenocarcinoma (n = 1), Non-Hodgkin lymphoma (n = 1). Maximum aspirated volume was 70 ml.

Conclusions: The aspiration of pancreatic mass can provide tissue material for the diagnosis of malignancy, combined CEA+CA19-9 and cytology studies enhanced diagnostic sensitivity for 38% (in comparison with single time aspiration cytology). EUS-FNA algorithm helps in the risk analysis leading for the medical, or surgical approach.

Miscellaneous

139

Delayed Gastric Emptying and Intestinal Hormones following Pancreatoduodenectomy

L. Strömmer[1], S. Räty[3], R. Hennig[4,5], T.E. Adrian, H. Friess[4], Y. Böttiger[2], J. Stanaitis[6], I. Nordback[3], J. Sand[3], U. Arnelo[1]

[1]Center for Surgical Sciences, [2]Dept. of Clinical Pharmacology, Karolinska Institutet at Karolinska University Hospital Huddinge, Stockholm, Sweden; [3]Dept. of Gastroenterology and Alimentary Tract Surgery, Tampere University Hospital, Tampere, Finland; [4]Dept. of Visceral and Transplantation Surgery, Heidelberg University Hospital, Heidelberg, Germany; [5]Northwestern University Feinberg School of Medicine, Chicago, Illinois, USA; [6]Dept. of Hepatology, Gastroenterology and Abdominal Surgery, Vilnius University Hospital, Vilnius, Lithuania

Introduction: Delayed gastric emptying is frequently reported in patients following pancreatoduodenectomy (PD). The present study tested the hypothesis that gastrointestinal hormones known to effect gastric emptying contribute to delayed gastric emptying in patients after PD.

Methods: Patients with (delayed, n = 9) or without clinical signs of delayed gastric emptying (non-delayed, n = 22) after PD were investigated. Plasma concentrations of motilin, glucagon-like peptide-1 (GLP-1), neurotensin, and peptide YY (PYY) and the gastric emptying rate (GER), assessed by the paracetamol absorption method were measured after a liquid meal on the 11th postoperative day.

Results: Days with a nasogastric tube ($p < 0.01$), days until solid food was tolerated ($p < 0.05$), and hospital stay ($p < 0.001$) were increased in delayed compared to non-delayed patients. The integrated peptide responses of motilin and GLP-1 were similar, but the responses of neurotensin and PYY were reduced, in delayed compared to non-delayed/normal patients, whether considered on clinical grounds or by measured GER ($p < 0.05$–0.005).

Conclusion: Neurotensin and PYY have both been shown to slow the rate of gastric emptying in humans. Therefore, these findings suggest that the reduced hormone responses were a consequence, rather than a cause, of delayed gastric emptying and thereby, delayed delivery of nutrients to the distal intestine, where the endocrine cells producing neurotensin and PYY are localized.

140

Postprandial Blood Glucose Control and Pancreatic Exocrine Function in Health and Diabetes Mellitus

J. Keller, S. Brueckel, A. Gresens, C. Jahr, C. Fibbe, P. Layer

Israelitic Hospital, University of Hamburg, Germany

Background: In healthy humans, increased postprandial blood glucose concentrations are known to contribute to regulation of gastrointestinal functions, specifically to the inhibitory control of gastric emptying (GE). By contrast, their effects on pancreatic exocrine secretion in health and diabetes mellitus are unknown. Thus, we investigated whether in healthy subjects or diabetics with normal GE pancreatic exocrine function is associated with blood glucose control.

Methods: 10 healthy subjects and 11 diabetics (7 type I, 4 type II, HbA1c 8.2 ± 0.3%, mean ± SE) with normal GE measured by ^{13}C-octanoic acid breath test ($T1/2 < 200$ min) underwent a secretin-cerulein test (SC-test) and a ^{13}C-mixed triglyceride breath test (MTG-BT) for direct and indirect measurement of pancreatic exocrine function. Tests were performed on separate days and after diabetic patients had taken an adequate morning dose of insulin/oral antidiabetics. Blood glucose was measured at 30 min intervals during both tests and only corrected by i.v. glucose or s.c. insulin if it was below 60 or exceeded 350 mg/dl, respectively.

Results: In diabetics, maximal blood glucose concentrations were higher than in controls during both tests (SC-test: 134 ± 8 vs. 97 ± 5 mg/dl, MTG-BT: 205 ± 7 vs. 113 ± 6 mg/dl, $p < 0.003$). Moreover, diabetics had decreased pancreatic exocrine function, both, measured by SC-test (amylase: 308 ± 37 vs. 525 ± 60 U/min, $p = 0.005$) and MTG-BT (cumulative 6-h-^{13}C-exhalation: 25 ± 2 vs. 37 ± 4% of dose, $p = 0.003$). In healthy subjects mean postprandial blood glucose was directly correlated with cumulative ^{13}C-exhalation ($R = 0.63$, $p < 0.05$). By contrast, in diabetics blood glucose and pancreatic exocrine function were not correlated, neither during MTG-BT ($R = 0.34$, NS) nor during SC-test ($R = 0.48$, NS).

Conclusions: Postprandial blood glucose and pancreatic exocrine responses are correlated in health but not in diabetes. Pancreatic exocrine function is reduced in diabetics, even in those without evidence of autonomic neuropathy as suggested by normal gastric emptying.

141

Sonographic Diagnostics of Pancreas Adipose Dystrophy in Combined Alcoholic Pathology of Pancreas and Liver

N.B. Gubergrits, E.V. Lobas

Chair of the Internal Diseases, Donetsk State Medical University, Ukraine

Introduction: Long-term alcohol abuse is a cause of combined liver and pancreas lesion. Initially fatty hepatosis and adipose dystrophy of pancreas develop, then – chronic steatohepatosis and chronic alcoholic pancreatitis (CAP). We performed our research to work out sonographic criteria for differentiation of pancreas adipose dystrophy and CAP.

Methods: 86 patients with combined alcoholic lesion of liver and pancreas were observed in our clinic. For differentiation of CAP and pancreas adipose dystrophy we used ultrasound histography (apparatus ALOKA SSD 630), which was conducted in region of pancreatic head. We took in to consideration histographic index L, which is obtained automatically during ultrasound histography, index of homogeneity (N) and histographic coefficient (K_{gst}), which are calculated with the help of original formulas worked out in our clinic.

Results: A subjective assessment of pancreas sonography did not allowed to differentiate CAP and pancreas adipose dystrophy, as moderate enlargement of pancreas and increasing of its echogeneity were revealed in both cases. Histographic index L was elevated in both cases as well, because it reflects tissue echogeneity. But CAP is characterized by heterogeneity of pancreatic tissue, so index N decreased to 3.4 ± 0.3%, its normal level – 5.2 ± 0.5% ($p < 0.05$). In case of pancreas adipose dystrophy the process was diffuse and homogenous, so N did not differ reliably from the normal level and amounted 4.9 ± 0.2%. K_{gst} was normal too in pancreas adipose dystrophy and significantly decreased in CAP – 30.7 ± 4.3 (in healthy – 122.4 ± 12.3, $p < 0.05$). With the help of ultrasound histrography we could diagnose CAP in 56 of the patients, pancreas adipose dystrophy – in 30 another patients. Therapeutic tactics was diagnose-dependent.

Conclusion: Ultrasound histography is an informative method in differential diagnostics of pancreas adipose dystrophy and CAP.

142

Changes in Nitric Oxide (NO) System and their Correction in Pancreas Pathology on the Background of Abdominal Ischemic Syndrome

N.B. Gubergrits, N.G. Agapova

Chair of the Internal Diseases, Donetsk State Medical University, Ukraine

Introduction: Atherosclerosis of abdominal aorta, celiac trunk, superior and inferior mesenteric arteries lead to development of abdominal ischemic syndrome resulted in inadequate blood supply of digestive organs including pancreas. We studied clinical peculiarities of pancreas lesion and NO metabolism in patients with atherosclerosis of abdominal aorta and its branches to work out methods of treatment.

Methods: 60 patients with pancreas lesion on background of abdominal ischemia were examined in our clinic. All patients were older than 60 years. For diagnose confirmation we used dopplerography of aortic branches, sonography of pancreas. Blood concentration of NO metabolites – nitrates and nitrites (labkits RD Systems, USA) – was assessed in all patients. 30 healthy persons were also examined.

Results: Clinical peculiarities of patients with pancreas lesion on the background of abdominal ischemia were the follow: dependence of pain syndrome from meal amount, rather than its type; ineffectiveness of spasmolytics and low response on analgesics; uncertain pain localization (not in left hypochondrium, but in meso-, epigastrium). Excretory pancreatic insufficiency progressed quickly in these patients; the level of the fecal elastase-1 was 62.3 ± 2.4 μg/g. Nitrate/nitrite blood level in patients was 3.12 ± 0.21 μmol/L that is reliably lower than the normal (in healthy subjects – 5.27 ± 0.36 μmol/L). The treatment scheme was supplemented with preparation on the basis of arginine glutamate (Glutargin). After the treatment clinical manifestations decreased; NO metabolites blood level increased significantly up to 4.26 ± 0.14 μmol/L.

Conclusion: Metabolic disorders in system of NO play an important role in pathogenesis of pancreas pathology on the background of atherosclerosis of abdominal aorta and its branches. It is recommended to include arginine glutamate in the treatment of the disease.

143

Endoscopic Transpapillary Stenting of the Pancreatic Duct. A Scottish and Polish Experience

P.M. Brennan[1], T. Stefaniak[2], D. Dymecki[2], M. Dobosz[3], Z. Sledzinski[2], R.W. Parks[1]

[1]Department of Surgical Sciences, University of Edinburgh, UK; [2]Department of General, Endocrine and Transplant Surgery, Medical University of Gdansk, Poland, [3]Department of Gastroenterological Surgery, City Hospital, Gdynia, Poland

Introduction: Endoscopic retrograde cholangio-pancreatography is used in the diagnosis and management of many pancreato-biliary conditions. Specifically, this study aimed to assess the utility and outcome, in two specialist centres, of the increasing use of endoscopic trans-papillary pancreatic duct stenting to treat disruption or stenosis of the pancreatic duct.

Methods: Data was analysed from two supraregional specialist pancreatico-biliary centres in the UK and Poland, between January 1998 and August 2004.

Results: 44 endoscopic transpapillary pancreatic duct stenting procedures were performed in 40 patients (28 male, 12 female), with a median age of 46.6 years (range: 28–93 years). The median follow-up was 45 months (range: 5–78 months). The indications were pancreatic ascites (16 patients, 40%), pancreatic pseudocyst (8 patients, 20%), pancreatic duct stenosis secondary to chronic pancreatitis (7 patients, 18%), pancreatico-pleural fistula (4 patients, 10%), and pain (5 patients, 13%). Average duration of stent insertion for stenosis was 38 weeks, and for duct disruption 6 weeks. Successful resolution of duct disruption was achieved in 21 of 28 patients (75%). However, 2 patients required surgical intervention and 2 required other endoscopic stenting procedures. Pain resolved in 4 of 12 patients (33%) who had a pancreatic stent inserted for pain control. Four patients with pain secondary to chronic pancreatitis required surgical intervention.

Conclusion: Endoscopic trans-papillary pancreatic duct stenting is a valuable option for managing patients with pancreatic duct disruption. It has a further role in providing analgesia in selected patients with proximal pancreatic duct stenosis, although definitive surgery appears to provide better long-term management.

144

The Value of Somatostatin and its Analogues in Reducing Complications Associated with Pancreatic Surgery: A Meta-Analysis

N. Alexakis[2], S. Connor[1], O.J. Garden[1], E. Leandros[2], J. Bramis[2], S.J. Wigmore[1]

[1]Clinical and Surgical Sciences (Surgery), University of Edinburgh, Royal Infirmary, Edinburgh, UK; [2]First Department of Propedeutic Surgery, University of Athens School of Medicine, Athens, Greece

Aim: The role of somatostatin or its analogues in reducing complications following pancreatic resection is controversial. The aim of this study was to perform a meta-analysis on the available evidence to determine its benefit.

Method: A literature search using Medline and ISI proceedings with exploration of the references identified 22 studies. Of these, 10 met the inclusion criteria for data extraction. Estimates of effectiveness were performed using a fixed and random effects model. The effect was calculated as an Odds ratio with 95% confidence interval (OR (95%CI)) using the Mantel-Haenszel method. Level of significance was set at $p < 0.05$.

Results: A total of 1918 patients were compared. Somatostatin or its analogues did not reduce the mortality following pancreatic surgery (OR 1.17 (0.7–1.9), $p = 0.545$) but did reduce both the total morbidity (OR = 0.62 (0.46–0.85), $p = 0.003$) and pancreatic specific complications (OR 0.56 (0.39–0.81), $p = 0.002$). At low volume centres (<10 resections/year) somatostatin or its analogues were beneficial in reducing the incidence of pancreatic specific complications (OR = 0.42 (0.32–0.55), $p < 0.001$) but at high volume centres this effect disappeared (OR = 0.99 (0.58–1.68), $p = 0.96$). Somatostatin or its analogues reduced the rate of biochemical fistula (OR = 0.45, (0.33–0.61), $p < 0.001$) but not the incidence of clinical anastomotic disruption (OR = 0.80, (0.44–1.44), $p = 0.46$).

Conclusion: Somatostatin or its analogues would appear to be beneficial in reducing the incidence of complications following pancreatic surgery. This effect may be negated by high volume centres where lower overall rates of complications are reported. Whether a selective policy can be implemented requires further investigation.

145

Performance of Helical CT Scan in the Detection of Endocrine Tumours of the Pancreas and Duodenum

K. Nahon-Uzan[1], D. O'Toole[1], O. Hentic[2], M.-P. Vullierme[2], A. Aubert[1], L. Palazzo[1], V. Vilgrain[2], A. Sauvanet[1], J. Belghiti[1], P. Lévy[1], P. Ruszniewski[1]

[1]Medical-Surgical Federation of Hepato-Gastroenterology, [2]Department of Radiology[2] Beaujon Hospital, AP-HP, University of Paris VII, Clichy, France

Introduction: Endocrine tumours of the pancreas and duodenum (ET-PD) are often difficult to localise. Conventional CT scan offered moderately accurate detection in cases of small lesions (~40%). No study has addressed diagnostic precision of CT since the advent of helical CT scanning.

Aim: Evaluate the diagnostic precision of helical CT in the detection of ET-PD and involved adjacent lymph nodes compared to echoendoscopy (EUS) and somatostatin receptor scintigraphy (SRS).

Methods: Forty-eight patients between 1995–2004 with ET-PD who underwent surgery were included. All patients had pre-operative helical CT and EUS performed. SRS was available for 42 patients. Diagnostic precision of each examination was compared to the pathology results for the following tumour characteristics: localisation, number of lesions, size, and involved adjacent lymph nodes.

Results: Fifty-three primitive tumours were found at histology examination (5 patients had 2 primary tumours). Tumours were non-functional (n = 37) and functional (n = 16) with the following primary sites: pancreatic in 45 cases and duodenal in 8. Median size of the primary tumour was 15 mm (8–0) and 7 were < 20 mm (median size for pancreatic lesions: 25 mm (6–150); 18 were < 2 cm). CT correctly identified 46/53 (87%) tumours. Performance was slightly better for EUS (49/53; 92%) although not significantly different. The 7 tumours not seen at CT were <10 mm in size. SRS did not detect lesions not seen on either CT or EUS (diagnostic precision: 69%). Node-positive disease was confirmed in 12 patients and was pre-operatively detected by CT and EUS in 5 and 6 cases, respectively.

Conclusion: In the detection of ET-PD the performance of CT has been impressively enhanced with helical acquisition and its diagnostic precision is similar to EUS (with the exception of very small lesions (< 10 mm)). Spiral CT can thus be proposed as a non-invasive first-line procedure in patients with a suspicion of ET-PD.

146

Prognosis of High Ki-67 in Well-Differentiated Metastatic Gastro-Entero-Pancreatic (GEP) Tumours

O. Hentic[1], D. O'Toole[1], A. Couvelard[2], K. Nahon-Uzan[1], O. Corcos[1], J.M. Tigaud[1], P. Hammel[1], P. Lévy[1], P. Ruszniewski[1]

[1]Medical-Surgical Federation of Hepato-Gastroenterology, [2]Department of Pathology, Beaujon Hospital, AP-HP, University of Paris VII, Clichy, France

Introduction: Well differentiated GEP tumours have a better prognosis than poorly-differentiated tumours, the latter have a high cellular proliferative index, Ki-67 (≥15%). Ki-67 levels varied in well-differentiated GEP from < 5% to 15%. Clinical significance of high Ki-67 levels (≥10%) in well-differentiated tumours remains unknown.

Aim: Determine prognosis in metastatic well-differentiated GEP with a high Ki-67 (≥10%).

Patients and Methods: Patients with GEP (06/94–03/04) respectively included and separated into 3 groups according to histology (WHO 2000) and Ki-67 scores: group A (well-differentiated, Ki-67 < 10%), group B (moderately-differentiated or well-differentiated, Ki-67 ≥ 10%), group C (poorly-differentiated, Ki-67 ≥ 15%). Other factors studies were: site of primary tumour, treatment and survival (Kaplan-Meier).

Results: 49 patients were included (A, n = 20; B, n = 15; C, n = 14). The sex ratio and median age were equally distributed in the 3 groups. The origin of the tumours was pancreatic in 40% (A), 67% (B) and 50% (C) of cases (NS). All patients had liver metastases and extra-hepatic metastases were observed in 20%, 40% and 21% of groups A, B and C, respectively (NS). In group C, 13 of 14 patients (92%) were treated using VP16-cisplatin as 1st-line with OR or stabilisation in 5 (38%) for 4 months. In group B, 9 of 15 patients received VP16-cisplatin (3 as 1st-line) with OR or stabilisation in 55%. Survival correlated with tumour type and percentage deaths were: 5, 33 and 64% for groups A, B and C, respectively. Concerning survival, group B have an intermediate prognosis compared to groups A and C (Log Rank test; $p < 0.0001$).

Conclusion: Prognosis in metastatic GEP depends on tumour differentiation but also on Ki-67 level. Well-differentiated GEP with high Ki-67 have a poor prognosis approaching that of poorly-differentiated tumours. Response to VP16-cisplatin also underlines the similar biological behaviour between well- or moderately-differentiated GEP with high Ki-67 and their poorly differentiated counterparts.

147

Quantitative mRNA Expression of Somatostatin (sst2, sst3, sst5) and Dopamine D2 Receptors in Pancreatic and Digestive Endocrine Tumours

D. O'Toole[1], A. Saveanu[2], A. Couvelard[3], G. Gunz[2], A. Enjalbert[2], P. Jaquet[2], P. Ruszniewski[1]

[1]Service de Gastro-entérologie, Hôpital Beaujon, Clichy; [2]Laboratoire Interactions Cellulaires Neuroendocriniennes UMR 6544-CNRS, Faculté de Médecine Nord, Marseille, France

Introduction: Somatostatin (SS) receptors (sst) are present in the majority of GEP with a predominance of sst2 (>80%). Effects of SS analogues are partial and of limited duration. GEP cell lines express D2DR. New chimeric analogues simultaneously recognising sst2 and sst5 (BIM-23244, SOM-230), or sst2 and D2DR (BIM-23A387) have additive inhibition of GH and prolactin secretion in pituitary adenomas.

Aim: analyse and quantify co-expression of sst et D2DR in human GEP.

Patients and Methods: mRNA expression (sst2, sst3, sst5 and D2DR), using RT-PCR (Taqman) in a series of 35 patients with GEP (pancreas [n = 19], midgut [16]). Levels of expression were compared with pituitary adenomas.

Results: All GEP expressed mRNA (variable quantities) for both sst2 (0.74 ± 0.55 copy/copy mRNA βGus) and D2DR (0.50 ± 0.39). sst5 was identified in 28/34 GEP analysed (0.91 ± 0.79); sst3 in only 34%. Compared to pituitary adenomas, mean expression in GEP was 55% for sst2, 9% for D2DR and 11% for sst5. However, high receptor levels similar to that of pituitary adenomas were found in 56% of GEP for sst2, 26% for D2DR and 24% for sst5. Expression of sst2 and D2DR was similar for pancreatic or midgut GEP; pancreatic GEP more frequently expressed sst5 ($p = 0.05$). Mean sst2 and D2DR expression (mRNA [copy/copy] x100) correlated with tumour aggressivity (121 vs. 42 for sst2 in WHO stage II and III GEP tumours, respectively [$p = 0.04$]; and 88 vs. 23 for D2DR in stages II and III, respectively [p = 0,03]).

Conclusions: 1) GEP co-express sst2 and D2DR in 100% of cases and sst5 in 80%. 2) Mean level of receptor expression especially for sst5 and D2DR is lower than in pituitary adenomas. 3) Advanced tumour WHO stage is associated with loss of sst2 et D2DR. 4) In vitro testing of bi-specific agonists is warranted in GEP tumours.

148

Role and Indications of Fluorodeoxyglucose Positron Emission Tomography (FDG-PET) in Neuroendocrine Pancreatico-Duodenal Tumors

C. Pasquali[1], C. Sperti[1], S. Scappin[1], C. Lunardi[1], F. Chierichetti[2], G. Liessi[3], S. Pedrazzoli[1]

[1]Clinica Chirurgica IV, Medical and Surgical Science Department, University of Padova; [2]Nuclear Medicine and [3]Radiology, Castelfranco Veneto Hospital, Italy

Introduction: Neuroendocrine pancreatico-duodenal tumors (NPDT) detection by imaging is a problem. PET provides biochemical and functional information on several tumors. Few studies reported the ability of FDG-PET to differentiate benign from malignant NPDT. Aim of this study was to evaluate the role of FDG-PET and to assess its indications in patients with NPDT.

Methods: From 1994 to 2004, 70 patients 33 male and 37 female, (mean age 52.2 years, range 18–84) with NPDT (82.85% pancreatic) were investigated with FDG-PET. PET results were compared with CT-scan, MRI and Octreoscan scintigraphy and clinico-pathologic features of patients and survival.

Results: Overall PET sensitivity was 55.7%; 79% of malignant tumors, and 17% of benign tumors were detected by FDG-PET. No duodenal tumor was detected by PET scan. Only 16% of primary less than 2 cm in size was localized. In 17.9% of cases PET scan provided new informations able to change therapeutic management. In PET positive patients the addictive informations obtained by PET scan when compared with Octreoscan, MRI and CT scan were respectively 40.5% more, 21.7% more and 25.6% more. In malignant neuroendocrine tumors PET positivity was related to short survival. No patient with malignant tumor died for disease progression in the follow-up when PET was negative, while 13/30 PET positive patients died ($p < 0.03$).

Conclusions: FDG-PET proved to be a second line technique in neuroendocrine pancreatico-duodenal tumors. PET results improve clinical staging of disease and is related to survival in malignant cases; in 17% of cases may change the therapeutic option. From our experience FDG-PET should be reserved for patients with suspected malignant tumor or pancreatic mass more than 2 cm or MEN I cases with at least one visible lesion. PET is not useful in duodenal tumors, benign insulinomas and small single pancreatic neuroendocrine lesion.

149

The Impact of Endoscopic Versus Surgical Approach on the Treatment Outcomes of Pancreatic Pseudocysts

E. Zdanyte, K. Strupas, S. Jurevicius, A.Sileikis

Centre of Abdominal Surgery, Vilnius University Hospital "Santariskiu Klinikos", Vilnius, Lithuania

Introduction: The introduction of minimally invasive techniques has increased the options for the management of pancreatic pseudocysts

(PPCs). Endoscopic drainage has provided a good alternative to a surgical treatment of PPCs. Surgical approaches allow a wide and permanent internal decompression, resection of PPCs together with the underlying diseased pancreas as necessary. The purpose of our study was to evaluate the impact of endoscopic versus surgical management, etiological and morphological peculiarities of PPCs and underlying pancreatic pathology on the treatment outcomes.

Methods: 106 patients, mean age 44.9 years (range, 20–87) with symptomatic and/or bigger than 5 cm PPCs were managed by endoscopic or/and surgical approach from 2000 to 2004. Data regarding clinical presentation, etiology and morphological characteristics of PPCs, pancreatic head and duct pathology, operative procedures were collected prospectively.

Results: 39 patients with 40 PPCs underwent endoscopic drainage procedures: 15 wall incisions, 24 cases of transmural drainage with double pigtail stent, 1 pancreatic duct sphincterotomy. 29 (72.5%) PPCs completely resolved. 2 patients underwent emergency operation because of unsuccessful endoscopic haemostasis. 4 patients were operated in cases of free gastric wall perforation. 3 patients required subsequent operations because of infected parapancreatic necrosis, 2 because of insufficient PPCs drainage. 68 remaining patients had surgical procedures: cystojejunostomy (29), cystogastrostomy and cystoduodenostomy (1), pancreatic resection (21), external drainage (5), extirpation (3), pancreaticojejunostomy (9). The morbidity rate was 14.7%, postoperative mortality 1.5%. The PPCs recurrence rate was 5% and 2.9% in endoscopic and surgical group respectively.

Conclusions: Endoscopic drainage is an effective alternative to surgical treatment of PPCs. Surgical management is necessary in cases of PPCs without close opposition to gastrointestinal wall, pancreatic and/or parapancreatic necrosis, underlying pancreatic head enlargement and/or pancreatic duct stricture, duct cutoff or dilation (>6 mm) when pancreatic resection and/or duct drainage operations are indicated.

150

A Clinical Analysis of the Minimally Invasive Pancreatectomy without Lymphadenectomy for Intraductal Papillary-Mucinous Neoplasms (IPMNs)

N. Kanai[1], *T. Hatori*[1], *A. Fukuda*[1], *S. Onizawa*[1], *T. Imaizumi*[2], *K. Takasaki*[1]

[1]Department of Gastroenterological Surgery, Tokyo Women's Medical University, Tokyo, Japan, [2]Department of Gastroenterological Surgery, School of Medicine, Tokai University, Isehara, Japan

Background: Intraductal papillary-mucinous neoplasms (IPMNs) are a unique tumor, which grows slowly and has a favorite prognosis. The minimally invasive pancreatectomy without lymphadenectomy is sometimes performed in case of that IPMNs have dysplasia or non-invasive carcinoma. The aim of this study is to evaluate the operative results of the minimally invasive pancreatectomy for IPMNs.

Methods: A total of 217 patients who underwent pancreatectomy for IPMNs between 1980 and 2004 were retrospectively chosen in this study. Duodenum-preserving pancreatic head resection (DPPHR), spleen-preserving distal pancreatectomy (SPDP), middle pancreatectomy (MP) and partial pancreatectomy of the pancreatic head (PR) were classified as a minimally invasive pancreatectomy ($n = 47$) and they were compared with conventional pancreatectomy ($n = 170$) including pancreatoduodenectomy, pylorus-preserving pancreatoduodenectomy, distal pancreatectomy with spleen and total pancreatectomy.

Results: Lymph node metastases were seen in only invasive carcinoma. Dysplasia and non-invasive carcinoma were seen higher with 98% in minimally invasive pancreatectomy than 70% in conventional pancreatectomy($p < 0.05$). There were no differences in the operative time and blood loss between the groups. However, morbidity rates were higher with 23% in minimally invasive pancreatectomy than 11% in conventional pancreatectomy including pancreatic fistula. Tumor recurrence was seen in one patient who underwent minimally invasive pancreatectomy for the invasive carcinoma.

Conclusion: Minimally invasive pancreatectomy without lymphadenectomy should be performed for IPMNs with dysplasia or non-invasive carcinoma, but it is required to improve the operative procedure more safely.

Pancreatology

Author Index for Abstracts

Numbers refer to abstract number

KARGER

Fax +41 61 306 12 34
E-Mail karger@karger.ch
www.karger.com

Accessible online at:
www.karger.com/pan

Pancreatology

Pancreatology 2005;5(suppl 1):103–110
DOI: 10.1159/000086078

Published online: June 3, 2005

5th International Symposium on Inherited Diseases of the Pancreas

Selected Abstracts

July 9, 2005,
Graz, Austria

Guest Editors
Markus M. Lerch, Greifswald
Thomas Griesbacher, Graz
David C. Whitcomb, Pittsburgh, Pa.

KARGER

Basel · Freiburg · Paris · London · New York ·
Bangalore · Bangkok · Singapore · Tokyo · Sydney

A1

The Clinical Course of Hereditary Pancreatitis in Children

G. Oracz[1], *B. Oralewska*[1], *A. Sobczynska-Tomaszewska*[2], *M. Teisseyre*[1], *J. Ryzko*[1], *J. Bal*[2], *J. Socha*[1]

[1]Department of Gastroenterology, Hepatology and Immunology, The Children's Memorial Health Institute, Warsaw, [2]Department of Medical Genetics, National Research Institute of Mother and Child, Warsaw, Poland

Introduction: The etiology of chronic pancreatitis (CP) in children is varied. The reported pediatric experience with hereditary pancreatitis (HP) is small. The aim of this study was to evaluate the clinical aspects of HP in children.

Methods: 107 children with CP, hospitalized since 1995 to 2005, were enrolled into the study. The medical records of these patients were reviewed for data on the presentation, diagnostic findings and endoscopic treatment. All children were screened for gene mutations (PRSS1, CFTR, SPINK1) by direct DNA sequencing.

Results: PRSS1 gene mutations were found in 14 patients (13%) (12 girls and 2 boys; mean age 8.03 years, range: 2.7–16.2 years). We detected R122H/- in 7 patients, R122C/- in 5 patients and N29I/- in 2 patients. In 2 patients with HP we found pancreas divisum. In one patient we found SPINK1 mutation (N34S/-); hyperlipidemia was found in one other patient. Family history was positive in all children with HP. There was no difference in age of the disease onset between HP group and non-HP group (8.03 years vs. 9.0 years; NS). In all children with HP ERCP had evidence of CP (2 moderate and 12 severe-according to the Cambridge Classification System, mean 2.8° Cambridge grade vs. 1.8° in non-HP group; $p < 0.05$). Therapeutic intervention, including both surgical and endoscopic intervention, was more frequent in the HP group (85.7% vs. 51.6%; $p < 0.05$). Pancreatic duct stenting was done in 10 children with HP (71.4% vs. 25% in non-HP group; $p < 0.05$). Extracorporeal shock wave lithotripsy was performed more frequent in HP group (35.7% vs. 3.2% in non-HP group; $p < 0.05$).

Conclusions: (1) HP in children has worse clinical course than CP in children without PRSS1 mutations. (2) We should be aware of coexisting HP and other factors causing CP, as anatomic anomalies.

Support from research grant KBN 3PO5E 13223.

A2

Trypsinogen Isoforms in the Pancreas of Various Mouse Strains

T. Wartmann[1], *P. Makarov*[1], *B. Brandt-Nedelev*[1], *T. Kähne*[2], *M.M. Lerch*[3], *M. Sahin-Tóth*[4], *W. Halangk*[1]

[1]Division of Experimental Surgery, and [2]Institute of Experimental Internal Medicine, Otto-von-Guericke University Magdeburg, Germany, [3]Department of Gastroenterology, Endocrinology and Nutrition, Ernst-Moritz-Arndt-University Greifswald, Germany; [4]Department of Molecular and Cell Biology, Boston University, USA

Introduction: Trypsinogen activation is thought to play a critical role in the pathogenesis of acute pancreatitis. Human trypsinogen is expressed in three isoforms: PRSS1, 2 and 3. Recently we have shown that five isoforms are expressed in the mouse pancreas (NMRI strain). On the other hand, transgenic and knock-out mice of various genetic background are frequently used to study experimental models of pancreatitis. Here, we studied the expression of trypsinogen isoforms in the pancreas of different mouse strains during pancreatitis and in controls.

Methods: The pancreas of mice (strains NMRI, CD-1, FVB, C57BL/6J) was obtained from unstimulated (saline injections) and caerulein-treated animals (7 hourly i.p. injections of 50 μg/kg bw). From the homogenized pancreas a secretory granule fraction was enriched, and this protein extract was used for 2D-PAGE. After silver staining protein spots were excised, proteolytically cleaved, the resulting peptides analysed by MALDI-TOF mass spectrometry and the proteins identified using NCBI Protein databases. Trypsin activity was determined using the colorimetric substrate Z-GPR-pNA.

Results: All mouse strains exhibit a comparable pattern of trypsinogen isoforms consisting of trypsinogens 5, 7, 8, 9 and 20. In FVB mice trypsinogen 8 represented a minor component. In all strains trypsinogen 5 was practically absent from the pancreas in control animals, but was strongly expressed after caerulein stimulation. The appearance of trypsinogen 5 was paralleled by a trypsin activity with lowered inhibitor sensitivity against soybean trypsin inhibitor.

Conclusions: Our results demonstrate that mice express a different pattern and more variable trypsinogen isoforms in the pancreas than humans. Strain-dependent differences concern trypsinogen 8 and the expression level of trypsinogen 5 after supramaximal hormone stimulation. Due to its structural homology to human mesotrypsin and rat trypsin 4 trypsinogen 5 could be responsible for the SBTI-insensitive trypsin activity after supramaximal caerulein stimulation.

KARGER

Fax +41 61 306 12 34
E-Mail karger@karger.ch
www.karger.com

1424–3903/05/0057–0104$22.00/0

Accessible online at:
www.karger.com/pan

A3

Endoscopic Evaluation and Management of Hereditary Pancreatitis Patients

P. Simon, A. Müther, F.U. Weiss, J. Mayerle, M.M. Lerch

Department of Gastroenterology, Endocrinology and Nutrition, Ernst-Moritz-Arndt-University Greifswald, Germany

Introduction: Most patients with hereditary pancreatitis develop progressive chronic pancreatitis with disease specific complications. Only limited data on the role of ERCP in the diagnosis and treatment of patients with hereditary pancreatitis are available. The aim of our study was to characterize the ERCP findings in hereditary pancreatitis patients, to test the validity of ERCP in detecting early malignant lesions and to determine the role of endoscopic interventions in a tertiary endoscopic referral center over a 4 year period.

Patients and Methods: 30 patients with hereditary pancreatitis (R122H-, R122C-, N29I-mutations) underwent ERCP and endoscopic interventions were performed on 12 patients.

Results: According to the Cambridge Classification 83% of the patients had high grade pancreatic duct changes, 50% had duct stones and 16% had strictures of the pancreatic duct that may have been caused by malignant changes. 89% of patients who underwent therapeutic interventions (e.g. papillotomy, ESWL, stone extraction or stenting) ultimately demonstrated disease progression. None of the patients had developed pancreatic cancer.

Conclusion: In our limited cohort not a single patient's early pancreatic neoplasia was identified by ERCP and lesions suspicious for neoplasia were not confirmed by CT or histology. Endoscopic interventions do not appear to halt disease progression but some patients' symptoms may benefit.

A4

The Cumulative Handicap of *CFTR* Sequence Variants in Patients with Idiopathic Chronic Pancreatitis

K. Truninger[1], B. Steiner[2], S. Gallati[2], M.-P. Audrezet[3], C. Ferec[3], M. Gomez-Lira[4], G. Cavallini[5], H. Witt[6]

[1]Division of Gastroenterology, Cantonal Hospital Aarau, Switzerland, [2]Division of Human Genetics, Department of Pediatrics, Inselspital Berne, Switzerland; [3]INSERM U613, Génétique Moléculaire et Génétique Epidémiologique, Centre Hospitalier Universitaire Brest, France; [4]Section of Biology and Genetics, Department of Mother and Child, University of Verona, Italy, [5]Department of Surgical and Gastroenterological Sciences, University of Verona, Italy; [6]Department of Pediatrics, Humboldt University Berlin, Germany

Introduction: In patients with nonclassic cystic fibrosis (CF), such as idiopathic chronic pancreatitis (ICP), often only one mutation in the *CFTR* gene can be detected. We recently reported a highly significant association between the presence of single-nucleotide polymorphisms (SNPs) and increased skipping of exon 9 and 12 in patients with nonclassic CF (Steiner et al. Hum Mutat 2004;24: 120–129). We therefore hypothesised that subjects carrying SNPs may be at risk to develop ICP.

Methods: 138 patients with ICP and 394 healthy controls were screened for a minimum of 40 mutations, several SNPs (nonsynonymous M470V, synonymous 2694T/G and 4521G/A) and the polyvariant TGT-repeat in intron 8 of the *CFTR* gene.

Results: Mutations were found in 50/138 (36%) patients and in 43/394 (11%) controls ($p < 0.001$). There was no significant association between the aforementioned SNPs, the (TG)12(T)7-repeat and ICP. ICP risk was increased approximately 44-fold by having two mutations, 3-fold by having one mutation and 1.4-fold by having one of the SNPs or the (TG)12(T)7-repeat. Carrying a single mutation plus one of the SNPs or the (TG)12(T)7-repeat had an additive effect on pancreatitis risk, raising the odds for ICP to approximately 20. This additive risk effect was supported by the fact that both a mutation and a SNP or the (TG)12(T)7-repeat were found in 26/138 (19%) patients, but only in 7/392 (2%) controls ($p < 0.001$). Finally, this finding was confirmed by segregation analyses in several families.

Conclusions: The presence of SNPs in the *CFTR* gene, particularly in combination with a single mutation, is associated with an increased ICP risk. Individuals carrying a single mutation may therefore not be simply carriers, but have an increased risk to develop monosymptomatic CF disease, such as ICP, by the additional presence of SNPs.

A5

Mutational Analysis of the Activation Peptide in Human Cationic Trypsinogen

Z. Nemoda, M. Sahin-Tóth

Department of Molecular and Cell Biology, Boston University Goldman School of Dental Medicine, Boston, MA, USA

Introduction: Activation of human cationic trypsinogen occurs upon proteolytic cleavage of the Lys23-Ile24 peptide bond by enterokinase or trypsin (autoactivation). The tetra-aspartate sequence (Asp19–22) preceding Lys23 in the trypsinogen activation peptide serves as specific recognition motif for enterokinase and inhibits autoactivation. This dual function of Asp19–22 is supposed to facilitate physiological trypsinogen activation in the duodenum, while preventing premature activation inside the pancreas. Here we present a detailed functional analysis of the Asp19–22 sequence in the context of full-length cationic trypsinogen.

Methods: Each Asp residue within the Asp19–22 sequence was individually replaced with Ala (D19A, D20A, D21A and D22A) or Glu (D19E, D20E, D21E and D22E). To prevent the confounding effect of autoactivation in the enterokinase-mediated activation experiments, double-mutants were also made in which the catalytic Ser200 was changed to Ala. Recombinant human enterokinase was purchased from R&D Systems. Cationic trypsinogen mutants were expressed in *Escherichia coli* and affinity-purified. Trypsinogen activation was followed by trypsin activity assays and SDS-PAGE.

Results: Human enterokinase activated wild-type cationic trypsinogen or mutants D19A, D20A and D21A at identical rates, while activation of mutant D22A was about 3-fold decreased. Autoactivation of the D19A and D21A mutants was 2-fold increased relative to wild-type cationic trypsinogen, while the D20A mutant exhibited a 4-fold increase. Dramatically, a more than 100-fold increase in autoactivation was observed with the D22A mutant. Even the conservative D22E mutation stimulated autoactivation 8-fold, while mutants D19E, D20E and D21E autoactivated normally.

Conclusions: Enterokinase recognition and cleavage of the activation peptide involves only Asp22, with no apparent contribution from Asp19–21. In contrast, maximal suppression of autoactivation requires the entire tetra-Asp sequence, although Asp22 is also the primary determinant of this function. The strong conservation of the tetra-Asp sequence is best explained by evolutionary selection against premature trypsinogen autoactivation.

A6

Exclusion Mapping of the 4q32–34 Locus in 41 European FPC Families

J. Earl[1], R. Kress[2], L. Yan[1], N. Howes[1], J. Leslie[1], L. Vitone[1], H. Rieder[3], M. Sina-Frey[3], S.A. Hahn[4], D.K. Bartsch[5], J.P. Neoptolemos[1], W. Greenhalf[1]

[1]The Division of Surgery and Oncology, RLUH, Liverpool, UK; [2]Department of Medical Biometry and Epidemiology, and [3]Department of Clinical Genetics, Phillips University of Marburg, Germany, [4]Department of Internal Medicine, Ruhr University of Bochum, Germany, [5]Department of Surgery, Phillips University of Marburg, Germany

Background: Familial Pancreatic Cancer (FPC) is a rare autosomal dominant disease, the causative gene(s) of which is unknown. The locus, 4q32–34 has been identified in one large American kindred as a potential locus for a disease gene.

Patients and Methods: The European Registry of Hereditary Pancreatitis and Familial Pancreatic Cancer (EUROPAC) and the Nationale Fallsammlung Familiäres Pankreaskarzinom (FaPaCa) have recruited 168 families with pancreatic cancer. The 4q32–34 locus has been haplotyped in affected and unaffected individuals in 71 EUROPAC and FaPaCa families with no known causative mutation. 9 mapping pairs between D4S413 and D4S415 from section 13 of the Genethon map of chromosome 4. These mapping pairs define an allele and haplotypes are assigned to each individual. A Two-Point-LOD-Score-Analysis was performed for each of the 9 markers. The model assumed an age-dependent penetrance and used two risk classes to allow for anticipation, which we observed in our FPC families. High Mobility Group Box 2 (HMGB2), cyclophillin D (PPID), mortality factor 4 (MORF4) and testican 3 (SPOCK 3) genes have been sequenced in affected individuals or obligate carriers.

Results: A LOD score of less than −2 was taken to indicate no linkage. For each marker LOD scores for theta values equivalent to centimorgan distances were plotted against the relative centimorgan position of the other markers on 4q32–34. LOD-Scores only rose above −2 in a region covering the markers 1539 and 1597. We have sequenced candidate genes within this region in FPC patients. Potential disease causing mutations or nucleotide polymorphisms in these genes have not been identified.

Conclusion: Although we cannot exclude a role for 4q32–34 in some of the families, it is unlikely that a dominant disease mutation is present in this region in the majority of European families.

A7

Gene Conversion between Functional Trypsinogen Genes Associated with Chronic Pancreatitis

N. Teich[1], Z. Nemoda[2], W. Heinritz[3], H. Köhler[4], J. Mössner[1], V. Keim[1], M. Sahin-Tóth[2]

[1]Medizinische Klinik II, University of Leipzig, Germany; [2]Department of Molecular and Cell Biology, Boston University Goldman School of Dental Medicine, Boston, MA, USA; [3]Institut für Humangenetik, University of Leipzig, [4]Klinik mit Poliklinik für Kinder und Jugendliche, Friedrich-Alexander-Universität Erlangen, Germany

Introduction: Gene conversion – the insertion or substitution of genetic material from another gene – is recognized as the underlying cause of a growing number of genetic diseases. While in most cases conversion takes place between a normal gene and its pseudogene, here we report a rare occurrence of disease-causing gene conversion between two functional genes. Chronic pancreatitis in childhood is frequently associated with mutations of the cationic trypsinogen gene.

Methods: We have analyzed the cationic trypsinogen gene in 1106 patients with chronic pancreatitis.

Results: We identified a novel conversion event affecting exon 2 and the subsequent intron. The recombination replaced 288 nucleotides with the paralogous sequence from the anionic trypsinogen gene, and resulted in amino acid substitutions N29I und N54S at the protein level. Analysis of the recombinantly expressed N29I-N54S double cationic trypsinogen mutant revealed increased autocatalytic activation, which was solely due to the N29I mutation.

Conclusion: Thus, gene conversion between two functional paralogous trypsinogen genes can produce an unstable trypsinogen molecule and can predispose to chronic pancreatitis.

A8

Genetic and Biochemical Characterization of the E32del Polymorphism in Human Mesotrypsinogen

Z. Nemoda[1], N. Teich[2], C. Hugenberg[2], J. Mössner[1], M. Sahin-Tóth[1]

[1]Department of Molecular and Cell Biology, Boston University Goldman School of Dental Medicine, Boston, MA, USA; [2]Medizinische Klinik und Poliklinik II, Universität Leipzig, Leipzig, Germany

Introduction: Mesotrypsin is a minor pancreatic digestive enzyme that degrades dietary trypsin inhibitors in the gut. In this study, we tested the hypothesis that the E32del genetic variant of mesotrypsin might represent a risk factor for the development of chronic pancreatitis, as a result of enhanced degradation of pancreatic secretory trypsin inhibitor.

Methods: We screened 97 German patients with chronic pancreatitis of alcoholic etiology and 109 healthy controls for the presence of the E32del variant.

Results: Higher allele frequency of the E32del variant was detected in the control population (25.7% vs. 18.0%), but the difference was not significant (p = 0.062). Recombinant mesotrypsin-E32del exhibited normal catalytic activity, characteristic inhibitor-resistance and inability to activate pancreatic zymogens. Degradation of trypsin inhibitors was unaffected by the E32del genotype. Interestingly, mesotrypsinogen-E32del was biochemically distinguishable from mesotrypsinogen by its faster activation with bovine enterokinase, while activation by human enterokinase, trypsin or cathepsin B was unchanged.

Discussion: The results classify mesotrypsinogen-E32del as a frequent polymorphic variant, which is not associated with chronic alcoholic pancreatitis.

A9

The Angiotensin-Converting Enzyme Insertion/Deletion Polymorphism is not Associated with Alcoholic and Idiopathic Chronic Pancreatitis

T. Hucl[1], M.-L. Kylanpää[2], B. Künzli[3], M. Lempinen[2], A. Schneider[1], E. Kemppainen[2], H. Friess[3], M. Löhr[1], M.V. Singer[1], R.H. Pfützer[1]

[1]Department of Medicine II, University of Heidelberg, Mannheim, Germany; [2]Department of Surgery, Helsinki University Central Hospital, Helsinki, Finland; [3]Department of General Surgery, University of Heidelberg, Heidelberg, Germany

Introduction: Chronic pancreatitis is characterised by a relapsing or continuing inflammatory process of the pancreas leading to irreversible fibrosis. Reduction in Angiotensin-Converting Enzyme (ACE) activity has been shown to attenuate pancreatic stellate cell activation and pancreatic fibrosis. The ACE gene insertion/deletion (I/D) polymorphism in intron 16 accounts for nearly half the variation in serum ACE levels. Our aim was to determine the frequency of the I/D polymorphism in patients with chronic pancreatitis.

Methods: After obtaining informed consent, one hundred and twenty six patients with chronic pancreatitis of different origin (94 alcoholic, 32 idiopathic, 64 of German and 62 of Finnish origin) and 245 control individuals (154 of German and 91 of Finnish origin) were genotyped for the I/D polymorphism by polymerase chain reaction.

Results: The prevalence of ACE genotypes and alleles was similar in patients and control individuals. Furthermore, genotype and allele frequencies did not significantly differ between patients with alcoholic and idiopathic chronic pancreatitis.

Conclusion: The role of the Renin-Angiotensin System (RAS) in chronic pancreatitis remains to be clarified. While changes in serum angiotensin levels may be of importance for pancreatic fibrosis, variations of the I/D polymorphism of the ACE gene appear not to account for susceptibility for alcoholic or idiopathic chronic pancreatitis.

A10

Common HFE Mutations are not Associated with Chronic Pancreatitis

T. Hucl[1], M.-L. Kylanpää[2], B. Künzli[3], M. Lempinen[2], A. Schneider[1], H. Friess[3], M. Löhr[1], E. Kemppainen[2], M.V. Singer[1], R.H. Pfützer[1]

[1]Department of Medicine II, University of Heidelberg, Mannheim, Germany; [2]Department of Surgery, Helsinki University Central Hospital, Helsinki, Finland; [3]Department of General Surgery, University of Heidelberg, Heidelberg, Germany

Introduction: Homozygous C282Y mutations of the HFE gene cause hereditary hemochromatosis, an autosomal recessive disorder of iron metabolism that results in progressive accumulation of iron in a variety of organs. Heterozygosity of C282Y and H63D mutations in the hemochromatosis gene may impair iron metabolism, increase the susceptibility or modify the severity of chronic alcoholic and non-alcoholic liver diseases. Excessive iron induces oxidative stress which plays a key role in the pathogenesis of liver cirrhosis and chronic pancreatitis. The aim of our study was to determine the frequencies of C282Y and H63D mutations in the hemochromatosis gene in patients with chronic pancreatitis.

Methods: A total of 138 patients with chronic pancreatitis (98 men, 40 women, median age 51 (22–81) years, 93 alcoholic, 45 non-alcoholic chronic pancreatitis, 69 of German and 69 of Finnish origin), 278 healthy controls (186 of German and 92 of Finnish origin) and 92 alcoholics without chronic pancreatitis were enrolled. DNA was isolated from peripheral blood leukocytes and genotyping of the C282Y and H63D alleles was performed by restriction fragment length polymorphism using *RsaI* and *MboI*. Association analysis was done using contingency table analysis and the chi-square and Fisher's exact tests for genotype and allele frequencies.

Results: The frequencies of HFE genotypes and alleles did not differ between patients with chronic pancreatitis and controls. Furthermore, genotype and allele distribution was similar in patients with alcoholic chronic pancreatitis and alcoholics without chronic pancreatitis. Genotype and allele frequencies were not different between patients with alcoholic and non-alcoholic chronic pancreatitis.

Conclusions: Changes in iron metabolism caused by HFE mutations do not seem to play a role in the pathogenesis of chronic alcoholic and non-alcoholic pancreatitis.

A11

Relationship between Interleukin Genotype and Severity of Acute Pancreatitis

E. De Madaria[1], J. Martínez[1], B. Lozano[2], L. Sempere[1], J. Sánchez-Payá[3], M. Pérez-Mateo[1]

[1]Sección de Aparato Digestivo, [2]Servicio de Inmunología, [3]Servicio de Medicina Preventiva, Hospital General Universitario de Alicante, Spain

Introduction: Currently the circumstances that determine that an acute pancreatitis (AP) becomes severe are not known. Some interleukins (IL) are highly increased in serum of patients with severe AP. IL are inflammatory mediators. Differences on IL genetic encoding may determine the severity of AP.

Aims: To investigate the relationship between different genotypes of IL-1, IL-1 receptor antagonist (IL-1RA), IL-6 and Tumour Necrosis Factor beta (TNF-B) with severity and etiology of AP.

Methods: Patients with AP were included consecutive and prospectively. Severity of the disease was determined according to Atlanta classification. Blood samples were obtained and the following polymorphisms were determined by PCR: L-1 (IL-1b 3954, IL-1b 511), IL-6 (IL-6 174, IL-6 597), IL-1 RA (IL-1 RA VNTR) and TNF-B (TNF-B 250).

Results: Eighty-four patients were included, 21 (25%) of them with severe AP. Allelic frequency was (% allelic frequency in severe AP vs. mild AP): IL-1b 3954: C (85.7 vs. 95.2), T (33.3 vs. 28.6); IL-1b 511: C (100 vs. 95.2), T (42.9 vs. 58.7); IL-6 -174: C (42.9 vs. 55.5), G (95.2 vs. 82.5); IL-6 597: G (90.5 vs. 93.7), A (47.6 vs. 58.7); IL-1RA: Allele 1 (85.7 vs. 85.7), Allele 2 (57.1 vs. 61.9), Allele 3 (0 vs. 3.2), Allele 4 (4.8 vs. 0); TNF-B 250: A (95.2 vs. 96.8), G (23.8 vs. 41.3). None of them (including its different genotypes) were significantly associated with neither disease severity nor etiology of AP.

Conclusion: Polymorphisms of L-1 (IL-1b 3954, IL-1b 511), IL-6 (IL-6 174, IL-6 597), IL-1 RA (IL-1 RA VNTR) and TNF-B (TNF-B 250) are not associated to severity nor etiology of acute pancreatitis.

A12

A Genetic Study on Pancreatic Cancer in Italy

M. Del Chiaro[1], L. Bertacca[1], A. Zerbi[2], M. Falconi[3], A. Giovannetti[1], G. Cipollini[1], M.A. Caligo[1], U. Boggi[1], G. Bevilacqua[1], G. Casari[2], M. Polese[2], V. Civelli[2] B. Longoni[1], V. Di Carlo[2], P. Pederzoli[3], G. Cavallini[3], S. Presciuttini[1], F. Mosca[1]

[1]Regional Referral Center for Pancreatic Diseases, University of Pisa, [2]San Raffaele Hospital, Milan, [3]University of Verona, Italy

Introduction: It is estimated that 3–5% of all pancreatic cancer cases may be caused by germline mutations in known genes, though it is increasingly recognized that some families carry an inherited susceptibility for pancreatic cancer unrelated to any currently identified syndrome.

Methods: Family history of cancer and blood samples are collected from all incident cases with pancreatic ductal adenocarcinoma ascertained by three participating groups. Pedigrees are recorded in a centralized database. The anatomical distribution of the number of cancers among first and second-degree relatives was compared with the cumulative risks published by Italian Cancer Registries for the 0–64 years age group.

Results: The database currently includes families of 351 probands, 145 females (41%) and 206 males (59%), with mean age at diagnosis of 65.5 and 63.7, respectively; pancreatic cancer among first-degree relatives was reported in 25 families (7.1%), 3 including two affected relatives, corresponding to 2.8-fold the population risk of at age 65 yr and to 3.0-fold increase at age >75 yr. Familial aggregation of cancers at any site was highly significant; gastrointestinal and uterine cancers were present in large excess. To investigate the role of BRCA2 in susceptibility to pancreatic cancer, the following eligibility criteria were established, prior to starting the molecular analyses: the probands with at least one first-degree relative with pancreatic cancer, or with breast cancer if <60 years, even of second-degree if in the paternal line, were selected for mutational screening. About 15% of the families met these criteria. Among nine patients analyzed by full sequencing, a missense mutation not previously described was detected, and a pathogenic mutation was identified in a proband with strong family history of breast cancer.

Conclusions: The present study provides the foundations for investigating the genetic susceptibility to pancreatic cancer in Italy.

A13

Mitochondrial DNA (mtDNA) Mutations: New Insights for Pancreatic Cancer Diagnosis and Prognosis

P. Fogar[1], F. Navaglia[2], D. Basso[2], E. Greco[2], C. Sperti[1], C.-F. Zambon[1], A. Falda[2], A. Stranges[2], C. Pasquali[1], S. Pedrazzoli[1], M. Plebani[2]

Departments of [1]Medical and Surgical Sciences and of [2]Laboratory Medicine, University of Padova, Italy

Introduction: The D-loop region is the major control site for mtDNA expression because it contains the reading strand for origin of replication and promoters for transcription. Somatic D-loop mutations have implicated in the pathogenesis of cancers. Our aims were to: 1) compare germline and pancreatic cancer (PC) mtDNA D-loop sequence; 2) verify whether in the germline mtDNA D-loop region there is any specific sequence correlated with PC diagnosis and outcome.

Methods: Stomatic (tumor) and germline (blood) mtDNA D-loop sequence was obtained from 24 PC and from blood of 12 age-matched healthy controls. mtDNA sequence was compared with the Cambridge sequence (www.mitomap.org).

Results: Hot spot differences between tumor and germline mtDNA were found only in 3 patients. Among the numerous SNPs identified in our sequences, only 4 of them were unbalanced between PC and controls. These SNPs (CT16189, CT16519, AG73, CT152) were analysed by DHPLC in a larger series of patients, including 100 PC, 41 chronic pancreatitis, 87 controls and 19 pancreato-biliary tract tumors. The haplotype T at 16189 and C at 16224 was correlated with pancreatic adenocarcinoma in non smokers ($X^2 = 4.8$, $p < 0.05$), but not in smokers ($X^2 = 0.01$, p: ns). In male, not in female patients with PC the mtDNA 16519 T allele was correlated with diabetes mellitus ($X^2 = 7.98$, $p < 0.05$). PC patients without distant metastases and bearing this allele survived significantly lower (Log Rank test = 9.74, $p < 0.005$).

Conclusions: 1) Somatic mtDNA mutations of the D-loop occur rarely in PC. 2) T16189-C16224 haplotype enhances PC risk in the absence of cigarette carcinogens exposure. 3) mtDNA 16519 T allele favors the onset of diabetes mellitus in PC supporting the role of mitochondria in the pathogenesis of this metabolic alteration. 4) The role of this allele in worsening metabolism is probably the basis of its association with a worse prognosis in non metastatic PC.

A14

Copy Number of Chromosome 17 but not HER2 Amplification Predicts Clinical Outcome of Patients with Pancreatic Ductal Adenocarcinoma

N.H. Stoecklein[1,2,5], A.M. Luebke[1], A. Erbersdobler[3], W.T. Knoefel[1,5], W. Schraut[2], P.E. Verde[4], F. Stern[1], P. Scheunemann[1,5], M. Peiper[1,5], C.F. Eisenberger[1,5], J.R. Izbicki[1], C.A. Klein[2], S.B. Hosch[1,5]

[1]Chirurgische Klinik, Universitätsklinikum Hamburg-Eppendorf, Hamburg, Germany, [2]Institut für Immunologie, Ludwig-Maximilians-Universität München, Germany, [3]Institut für Pathologie, Universitätsklinikum Hamburg-Eppendorf, Hamburg, Germany, [4]Koordinierungszentrum für klinische Studien, Universitätsklinikum Düsseldorf, Germany

Background: To determine the frequency and the potential clinical use of HER2 (17q21) gene amplification and chromosome 17 aneusomy in pancreatic ductal adenocarcinoma.

Methods: Serial tissue sections of 50 resected PDAC were analyzed with chromogenic in situ hybridization (CISH) using locus specific HER2 probes and centromeric probes for chromosome 17. Centromeric probes for chromosome 7 and 8 were hybridized to confirm ploidy levels. Expression of HER2 protein was assessed by immunohistochemistry. Correlations of experimental findings with clinical and follow-up data were tested.

Results: The HER2 gene locus was frequently (24%) amplified in PDAC and the rate of overexpression (2+ and 3+) was 10%, but no prognostic significance was found. Copy number analysis of chromosome 7, 8 and 17 revealed disomic (40%), trisomic (36%) and hyper-tetrasomic (24%) tumors. Compared to patients with disomic tumors patients with hyper-tetrasomic tumors exhibited a significantly decreased relapse-free and overall survival (5.0 months versus 13.0 months, $p = 0.0144$ and 7.0 months versus 20.0 months, $p = 0.0099$, respectively). Multivariate analysis confirmed the independent prognostic significance of hyper-tetrasomy.

Conclusion: Here we show that tumor ploidy levels correlate with prognosis of PDAC patients indicating characteristic biological properties of PDAC with high chromosomal instability. In contrast, no prognostic influence on patient outcome was found for the amplification of the HER2 oncogene or p185HER2 overexpression. Therefore, evaluation of ploidy levels offers new opportunities for patient stratification in clinical trials and enables novel approaches to study the well-known aggressiveness of PDAC.

A15

The Founder Effect in N29I Mutations is Greater than in R122H Mutations of the Cationic Trypsinogen Gene

L. Vitone[1], W. Greenhalf[1], N. Howes[1], T. Wong[1], R. Mountford[2], V. Blake[2], J.P. Neoptolemos[1]

[1]Division of Surgery and Oncology, Royal Liverpool University Hospital, Liverpool, UK, [2]Molecular Genetics Laboratory, Liverpool Women's Hospital, Liverpool, UK

Introduction: It has been established that point mutations in the cationic trypsinogen gene (PRSS1) are associated with hereditary pancreatitis. The two most frequent point mutations are in exon 2 (N29I) and exon 3 (R122H). These mutations are found in diverse racial populations. Both mutations result in early onset pancreatitis. It is unclear whether these are ancient mutations or whether they have spontaneously occurred in multiple populations.

Methods: A PCR/RFLP approach was used to identify the neutral polymorphism D162D in exon 4 of PRSS1 by introduction of the FokI restriction site in the rare allele. Individuals with hereditary pancreatitis on the European Registry of Hereditary Pancreatitis (EUROPAC) were tested for the alleles of D162D. The R122H and N29I mutations were linked to either the frequent or rare polymorphism of D162D.

Results: The rare allele of D162D was linked to N29I in three families and the frequent allele was linked to N29I in one family. The rare allele was linked to R122H in four families and the frequent allele was linked to R122H in ten.

Conclusions: Both common mutations in PRSS1 are linked to both alleles of the D162D polymorphism. This represents two separate populations for both mutations which can be analysed in terms of genetic and environmental factors.

Pancreatology

Author Index for Selected Abstracts

Numbers refer to abstract number

KARGER

Fax +41 61 306 12 34
E-Mail karger@karger.ch
www.karger.com

Accessible online at:
www.karger.com/pan

Pancreatology

Guidelines for Authors

Submission
Manuscripts written in English should be submitted using the online submission website

www.karger.com/pan

or as e-mail attachment (the preferred word-processing package is MS-Word) to the Editorial Office:

pan@karger.ch

R. Urrutia, MD
c/o S. Karger AG
Editorial Office 'Pancreatology'
P.O. Box
CH–4009 Basel
Tel. +41 61 306 1356
Fax +41 61 306 1434

Conditions
All manuscripts are subject to editorial review. Manuscripts are received with the explicit understanding that they are not under simultaneous consideration by any other publication. Submission of an article for publication implies transfer of the copyright from the author to the publisher upon acceptance. Accepted papers become the permanent property of 'Pancreatology' and may not be reproduced by any means, in whole or in part, without the written consent of the publisher. It is the author's responsibility to obtain permission to reproduce illustrations, tables, etc. from other publications.

Rapid Communications
Manuscripts intended for rapid communication must present new findings of sufficient importance to justify their accelerated acceptance. Readers are invited to send their contributions to the address given under Submission. Manuscripts should follow the normal arrangement of research papers, including an abstract not exceeding 150 words. Rapid communications should not be more than four printed pages in length (including figures, tables and references). Rapid communications can only be accepted as they are or with minor modifications. Rejected manuscripts can only be reconsidered as regular papers. Review will be rapid, and once accepted, the paper will be included in the next planned issue.

Clinical Images
Clinical Images is a feature of 'Pancreatology' that wants to give the GI surgeon the possibility to share an exceptional clinical condition encountered during his or her daily work with fellow surgeons. Readers are invited to send their contributions to the address given under Submission. Images must be original, unpublished, high-quality black-and-white photographs. Each print should be labeled with the last names of the contributors and an arrow indicating the top of the image. The legend/short text should explain the uniqueness of the depicted and provide relevant clinical information including a short description of the patient's history, relevant physical and laboratory findings, clinical course, response to treatment (if any) and condition, or both. This text should not exceed 200 words. Contributors must provide the names, academic degrees, addresses, phone and fax numbers of the photographer, contributor, or both.

Special Requirements
1. Investigations Involving Human Subjects: 'Pancreatology' requires that investigations performed on human subjects have the prior approval of the institutional committee on human experimentation. Authors are required to submit a signed statement as to the date and details of the appropriate review. In countries where such mechanisms for approval do not exist, authors are required to submit a signed statement that the research was carried out in accordance with the Helsinki Declaration. A similar assurance is required to document that animal experimentation was performed under appropriate circumstances.

2. Statement for Authors Submitting Original Research or Case Reports: 'The enclosed manuscript ... (Title) ... has been approved by me as well as by the responsible authorities at the institute where the work has been carried out. I certify that none of the material in this manuscript has been published previously in any form and that none of this material is currently under consideration for publication elsewhere. This includes symposia and proceedings of meetings and preliminary publications of any kind except an abstract of 400 words or less.' (To be signed by all authors.)

3. The undersigned also confirm that they qualify for (co-)authorship according to the 'Uniform Requirements for Manuscripts' published in the guidelines of the 'International Committee of Medical Journal Editors' in 1988 as follows: Authorship credit should be based only on substantial contributions to (a) conception and design, or analysis and interpretation of data; (b) drafting the article or revising it critically for important intellectual content; and on (c) final approval of the version to be published. Conditions (a), (b), and (c) must all be met. Participation solely in the acquisition of funding or the collection of data does not justify authorship. General supervision of the research group is also not sufficient for authorship. Any part of an article critical to its main conclusions must be the responsibility of at least one author. Persons who have contributed intellectually to the article but whose contributions do not justify authorship may be named and their particular contribution described in the 'Acknowledgements'. Such persons must give their permission to be named.

Arrangement
Title page: The first page of each paper should indicate the title, the authors' names, the institute where the work was conducted, and a short title for use as running head.
NB: Authors wishing to preserve the phonetic meaning of diacritics (PubMed reduces diacritics to their root characters) must spell their names accordingly when submitting manuscripts (e.g. Müller should be Mueller).

Full address: The exact postal address of the corresponding author complete with postal code must be given at the bottom of the title page. Please also supply phone and fax numbers, as well as e-mail address.

Key words: For indexing purposes, a list of 3–10 key words in English is essential.

Abstract: Each paper needs an abstract of up to 200 words. It should be structured as follows:

Background/Aims:	What is the major problem that prompted the study?
Methods:	How was the study performed?
Results:	Most important findings?
Conclusion:	Most important conclusion?

Footnotes: Avoid footnotes.

Tables and illustrations: Tables and illustrations (both numbered in Arabic numerals) should be prepared on separate pages. Tables require a heading and figures a legend, also prepared on a separate page. For the reproduction of illustrations, good drawings and original photographs are preferred; slides may also be accepted; negatives or photocopies cannot be used. Due to technical reasons, figures with a screen background should not be submitted. When possible, group several illustrations in one block for reproduction (max. size 180 × 223 mm) or provide crop marks. On the back of each illustration, indicate its number, the author's name, and 'top' with a soft pencil. Electronically submitted b/w half-tone and color illustrations must have a final resolution of 300 dpi after scaling, line drawings one of 800–1,200 dpi.

Color illustrations: Up to 6 color illustrations per page can be integrated within the text at the special price of CHF/USD 660.00 per page. Color illustrations are reproduced at the author's expense.

References: In the text identify references by Arabic numerals [in square brackets]. Material submitted for publication but not yet accepted should be noted as 'unpublished data' and not be included in the reference list. The list of references should include only those publications which are cited in the text. Do not alphabetize; number references in the order in which they are first mentioned in the text. The surnames of the authors followed by initials should be given. There should be no punctuation other than a comma to separate the authors. Preferably, please cite all authors. Abbreviate journal names according to the Index Medicus system. (Also see International Committee of Medical Journal Editors: Uniform requirements for manuscripts submitted to biomedical journals. N Engl J Med 1997; 336: 309–315. www.icmje.org)

Digital Object Identifier (DOI)
S. Karger Publishers supports DOIs as unique identifiers for articles. A DOI number will be printed on the title page of each article. DOIs can be useful in the future for identifying and citing articles published online without volume or issue information. More information can be found at www.doi.org.

Examples
(a) Papers published in periodicals: Chatel J-M, Bernard H, Orson FM: Isolation and characterization of two complete Ara h 2 isoforms cDNA. Int Arch Allergy Immunol 2003;131:14–18.
(b) Papers published only with DOI numbers:
Theoharides TC, Boucher W, Spear K: Serum interleukin-6 reflects disease severity and osteoporosis in mastocytosis patients. Int Arch Allergy Immunol DOI: 10.1159/000063858.
(c) Monographs: Matthews DE, Farewell VT: Using and Understanding Medical Statistics, ed 3, revised. Basel, Karger, 1996.
(d) Edited books: DuBois RN: Cyclooxygenase-2 and colorectal cancer; in Dannenberg AJ, Dubois RN (eds): COX-2. Prog Exp Tum Res. Basel, Karger, 2003, vol 37, pp 124–137.

Proofs
Unless indicated otherwise, proofs are sent to the first-named author and should be returned with the least possible delay. Alterations made in proofs, other than the correction of printer's errors, are charged to the author.

Reprints
Order forms and a price list are sent with the proofs. Orders submitted after the issue is printed are subject to considerably higher prices.

KARGER

Fax +41 61 306 12 34
E-Mail karger@karger.ch
www.karger.com

The Guidelines for Authors are available at:
www.karger.com/pan_Guidelines

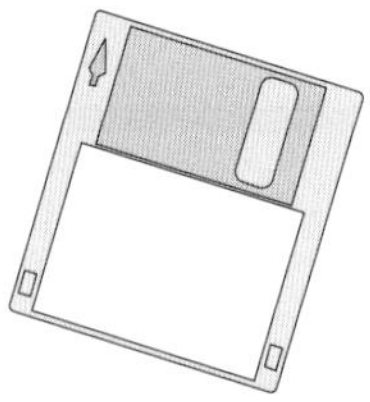

E-Mail and Disk Submission

A **comprehensive version** of these guidelines for e-mail and disk submission of manuscripts to 'Pancreatology' can be accessed online under **www.karger.com/disksubmission**

Style
Please follow the general rules on style and arrangement in the **'Guidelines for Authors'** of the journal.

Initial E-Mail or Disk Submission of Manuscripts
Manuscripts submitted to 'Pancreatology' should be sent as a single Word file (PC version) including the figures which must be placed at the end on separate pages, one figure per page. To avoid confusion, other formats will not be accepted at this stage. The manuscript may be e-mailed as an attached file or sent by mail on a 3.5-inch diskette.

Disk Submission of Final Version
Following acceptance for publication, authors will be requested to provide a disk (see below for specifications) with the final version of the manuscript. For this final version, text should be saved as a Word file, while figures should be in PowerPoint, both PC versions. The disk must be accompanied by two paper copies of the text and figures and a statement from the authors that the version is exactly the same as that which has been accepted.

a) Disk Format
Store only data pertinent to this manuscript. For a **text only** manuscript, use a 3.5-inch disk. For **text and illustrations,** use CD-ROM (DOS or hybrid) or iomega Zip/DOS (100 MB/250 MB).

b) Disk Description
Label your disk with the **title of the journal** for which it is submitted; a **short version** of the paper's title; your **name,** postal and e-mail address, fax and phone number; **hard and software** used, including the version; and the **complete list of the file names.** File names consist of eight characters before the dot identifying the file and three characters after the dot identifying the application.

c) Text Format
Enter your text continuously flush left. Do not use any layout functions. Do not split words at the end of a line. **Do not use indentations.** Use a blank line before and a hard return at the end of paragraphs. **Arrange headings flush left.** Insert only **one space after punctuation marks.** Insert Greek letters, mathematical symbols etc. with your word-processing program. Use **boldface and italics** as well as sub- and superscript where appropriate.

Tables are part of the text and should be placed at the end of the text file. Separate the individual parts of a table by lines. Use the tabulator instead of spaces. Format operation data on one line in the same column. **Legends to illustrations are part of the text** and should also be listed after the tables.

d) Illustrations
Store illustrations as separate files: do not integrate them into your text. Export **line drawings/vector graphics** as PowerPoint. Use Photoshop or similar software for processing and retouching **scanned half-tone images.** Save the original scan and the processed version. Export **black and white or color images** in PowerPoint format in their anticipated size in print. Illustrations should be submitted as PowerPoint files (PC version).

KARGER

Fax +41 61 306 12 34
E-Mail karger@karger.ch
www.karger.com

The Guidelines for Authors are available at:
www.karger.com/pan_Guidelines